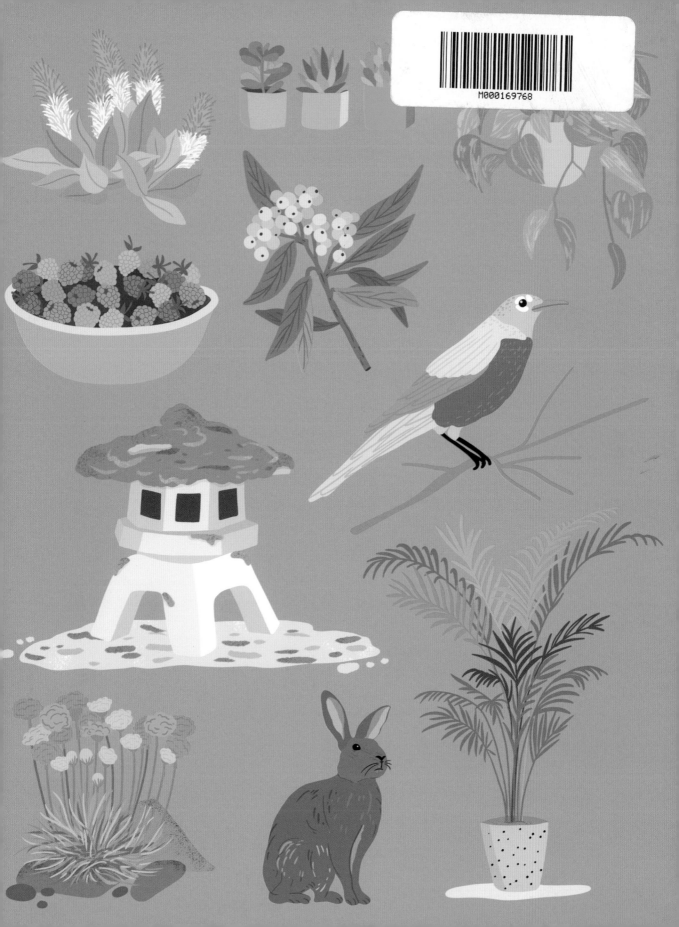

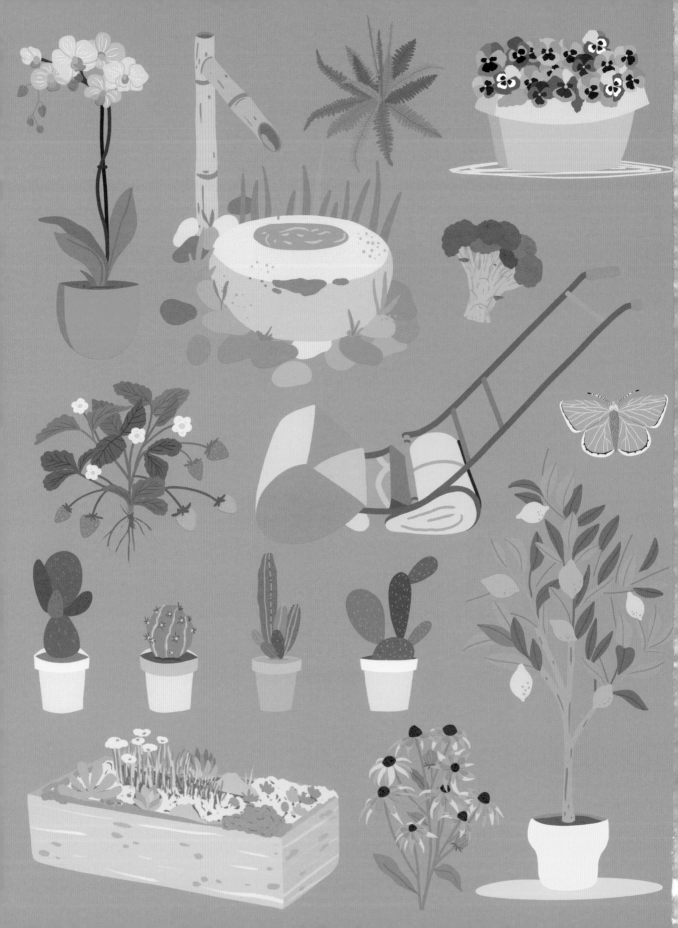

How Plants Can Save Your Life

50 INSPIRATIONAL IDEAS FOR PLANTING AND GROWING

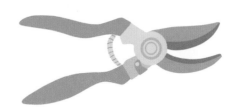

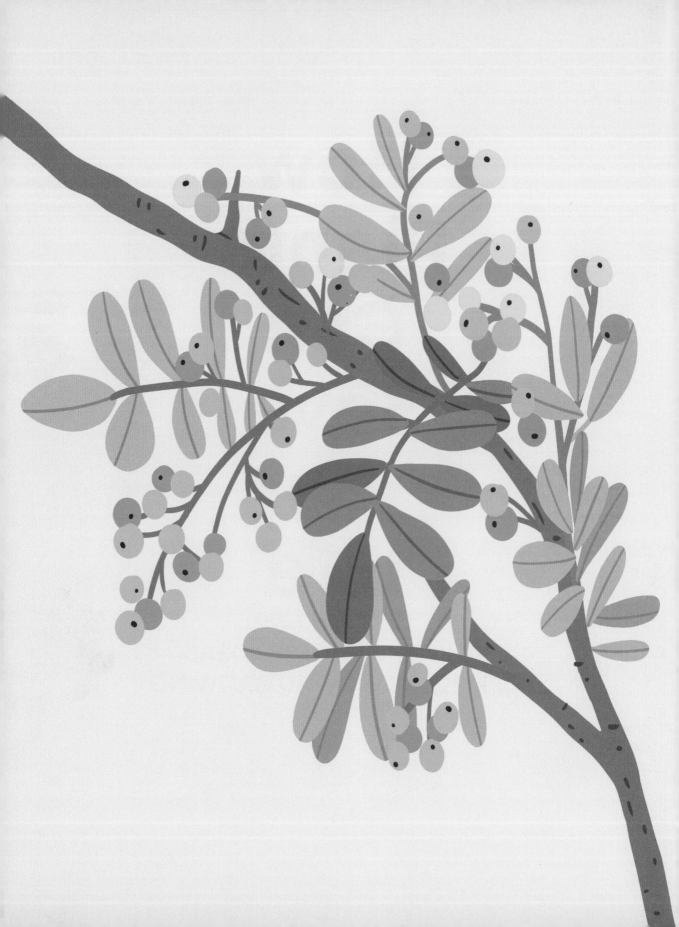

How Plants Can Save Your Life

50 INSPIRATIONAL IDEAS FOR PLANTING AND GROWING

DR ROSS CAMERON

greenfinch

Contents

Introduction 6

Nature and Well-being 8

Plants and Gardening: A Hobby, Not a Chore 10

50 Ideas and Health Benefits

Introduction

When I casually mention in conversation, 'Plants can save your life,' I get one of two distinct reactions from my listeners. Many folk shuffle uncomfortably, look at their watch and plan their escape from the deluded tree-hugger they have been so unfortunate as to bump into. The rest look me in the eye and ask, 'Just how much public money have you spent "proving" common sense?'

If you fall into the latter category, this book may not be for you. You already understand that our lives are dependent on plants; that we would not survive for more than two minutes without the oxygen they produce; that, because they are the basis of our food chain, we would starve after about a month without them; that they help to regulate the world's water, nutrient and even climate cycles, on which we depend; and – perhaps worst of all – you would die of embarrassment when you realized you were not wearing any clothes. So plants are vital, but this is not always recognized.

All these requirements are about the global relationships between plants and humans, however, and this book is actually about our intimate everyday relationships with plants. Even for the well-informed reader, I hope it will throw up a few surprises. The points I make are based on the latest research and touch on our increasing recognition of how valuable plants (and their allied organisms) are to the fundamentals of life, as well as to the quality of our individual lives.

> We depend upon nature for every breath we breathe and every mouthful of food we eat. And some people would say we depend upon it for our very sanity.
>
> *Sir David Attenborough*

When I first undertook research into the benefits of plants, in the late 1990s, I was astonished by just how widespread those benefits are. It is self-evident, of course, that plants are the fundamental component of a healthy diet, but I have subsequently been amazed at the way plant products and their allied microbes essentially administer this diet too. We require a healthy gut to digest our food, but also, importantly, to regulate our hormones, develop immunity to disease and protect our mental health (the so-called microbiota-gut-brain axis). Plant-based compounds and microbial communities found in nature directly encourage this fully functioning gut.

Moreover, we need green spaces if we are to relax and feel fulfilled, to experience the joy and wonder nature can bring. Exposure to plants can relax people within minutes. Street trees are now recognized by urban planners as crucial in allowing motorists to de-stress and to reduce tension in traffic jams. And we can get these benefits from just a few plants. In one study, my colleagues and I provided some non-gardeners with planted pots to place in front of their houses so that they would notice them as they entered and left. Over a number of weeks we observed that these people had significantly healthier levels of the stress hormone cortisol – indicating less chronic stress – than similar residents who had not been given plants. In the most extreme cases, providing views of and access to local green space has been linked to lower levels of domestic violence and even less gun crime. There are many ways a plant might save your life!

But plants do more than just make us relaxed. We think plants and the wild animals they draw in give people direct joy. Psychologists call these moments of joy 'positive affect' and, if repeated regularly, such moments build up resilience against poor mental health. Many gardeners acknowledge this. Finally, we should not forget the physical benefits plants bring to our homes and offices. They improve the quality of the air, disperse intrusive noise, keep us cool during heatwaves and lessen the risk of our homes flooding. This book highlights how we can use plants to optimize these significant and wide-ranging benefits.

Nature and Well-being

There is increasing evidence that a relationship with the natural world is vital for our health and well-being. We do not always have the time or resources to restore our vitality by escaping to the mountains or the seaside, but we can bring nature closer to us.

Growing plants and creating gardens (however small) can be fun, fascinating and a great way to explore and engage regularly with the natural world. What's more, it is good for our health. Gardening (and other forms of 'ecotherapy') can help to improve our mood, relax us, take us away from our everyday problems and promote positive emotions.

Being exposed to plants, cultivating them and taking part in garden activities have been linked to:

- reduced frequency or severity of depression
- reduced anxiety and stress
- delays in the onset of dementia
- increased feelings of joy
- improvements in physical fitness
- enhanced self-esteem
- better communication skills
- better diet

So why are plants and gardening good for you? There are a number of key concepts that explain our reaction to nature and the benefits we accrue from it. I explore these ideas in more detail later in this book, but to summarize, they are:

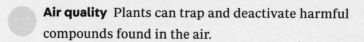 **Air quality** Plants can trap and deactivate harmful compounds found in the air.

Attention Restoration First put forward in 1989, this theory suggests that the natural world allows us to unwind by providing us with the capacity to escape from the source of our stress (Being away), to be distracted (Soft fascination) with features that we can engage with or be immersed in (Extent), and that we find interesting (Compatibility).

Biophilia We have an innate relationship with nature, where evolutionary processes determine how we perceive and respond to natural features.

Healthy eating By eating plant products, we ingest compounds that promote a healthy, balanced diet and regulate cell function.

Human microbiome Naturally occurring microbial communities influence our gut activity, and thus other aspects of our health.

Noise reduction Plants can muffle intrusive, stress-inducing noise.

Physical activity An interest in active outdoor pursuits keeps us physically fit.

Phytoncides (essential oils) Plants release these chemicals, which have anti-cancer and other beneficial properties, that we can absorb through forest bathing.

Positive affect Nature provides us with short bursts of happiness that improve our mental health.

Stress reduction Viewing green features affects our physiology and relaxes us.

Thermal comfort Plants shade and cool us during hot weather.

Plants and Gardening: A Hobby, Not a Chore

Plants are fun, and looking after them – gardening – can bring significant health benefits, but only if you see this activity in the right light. You will gain a great deal from interacting with plants, but it is best to view such interaction as a form of engagement and an opportunity for either activity or relaxation. Gardening can be hard work at times, but it should never be a chore. If you have become a slave to mowing the lawn, something is wrong. Think about the amount of time you have and garden according to that. If you already have a hectic life, adding plants but not freeing up time to enjoy them will just make your life even more frenetic.

To reap the health benefits of gardening, attitude is important. Challenge yourself by asking why you want to have houseplants, or to plant your garden space. It must be about you and your potential interests, not about 'keeping up with the Joneses' across the road. You should not do it because it is expected of you, or some sort of moral obligation. You should do it because you think you might enjoy it and that it might be fascinating to know more about your plants, or because you just want somewhere a bit more natural to sit in and relax.

A survey by the horticultural retail sector in 2011 suggested that a large proportion of people do not garden because of a fear of failure, or because they are anxious about being seen to fail by their peers or family. Despite what you see in media coverage of national flower shows, gardening should not be a contest. Or, if there is a competitive element, it should be about competing with yourself and in a fun way. If you are gardening, and gardening for well-being in particular, avoid the 'must-dos' you might be advised on, and instead adopt the 'like-to-dos'. This is about having fun.

Another reason newcomers avoid plants and gardening relates to knowledge. People do not want to be seen to be ignorant about plants – 'I don't know all the confusing long names'; 'I don't know when to prune my clematis'; 'I didn't want to look stupid in front of the garden centre staff.' Who cares about that? It is important to realize from the outset that you will have failures, but it's the trying that matters. Gardening is a journey – and an enjoyable and fulfilling one, I hope – but it's not an end point. The 'perfect' garden will still attract weeds.

You don't need to be an expert. Researching and knowing about plants can be fun, but it's not a requirement. What's the worst that can happen if you make a mistake? Apart from anything else, nature abhors a vacuum. So the prize rose died, but a whole lot of forget-me-nots came up instead. To enjoy gardening, and to reap the health benefits that come with it, you will find it helpful to develop a grounded attitude. This is about you working with nature, not controlling it, so there will be wins and losses.

This book gives some clues as to what you might plant, but these are only hints. Its main rationale is to inspire and give a few examples of what you can do. It's my intention to illustrate how these examples relate to our well-being, but the excitement is in the discoveries you will make for yourself. Be curious, explore, experiment, but most of all enjoy the 'journey' and relax in the new environs you create. That's the point, after all.

50 Ideas and Health Benefits

This book links benefits to health and well-being with specific plant-based activities. The idea is to provide an easy introduction to the wonderful world of plants for those who have not kept a houseplant, have never gardened or are yet to experience the beauty of a newly unfurled rose. For those who already have the 'plant bug', I hope this book will explain why you gain so much joy, satisfaction and relaxation from a session with your plants.

I have identified 50 ideas to encourage you to engage with plants and gardens. These are meant to strike an interest and be inspirational. The activities and types of plant chosen are deliberately diverse, to demonstrate that there should be something for everyone in terms of primary interest. Do note that these are not 'how to' guides; plenty of practical guides to plant cultivation are available. Rather, the objective is to show how working with plants or being in a garden can be restorative or provide enjoyment. Intermixed with the 50 activities are 'Health Benefit' sections, which outline the different ways plants influence our health and well-being. These sections provide the rationale of *how* plants provide these benefits to us and *why* we respond to them in the ways we do. Each of the 50 ideas links to one or more of the health benefits.

The book discusses easy activities, and I have chosen those that need not be time-consuming or expensive, but we must not underestimate the importance of such activities to our well-being. These are not luxuries or nice 'add-ons' to our lives, but fundamentally important to a healthy lifestyle.

It is clear that humans benefit immensely from engaging with plants and the natural world, but it is important to stress that this is an interrelationship. The natural world needs us to be onside for the sake of the health and well-being of the planet and its ecosystems. Plants allow us those first important steps, a tentative first touch to a wider natural world. If we love plants and gardens, we are much more likely to love the world's forests, its grasslands, its coral reefs. And when we love something, we care for it. For good or ill, the world's planetary systems are now in our hands, and we must understand, engage with, appreciate and – vitally – care for them. Plants are a really great place to start.

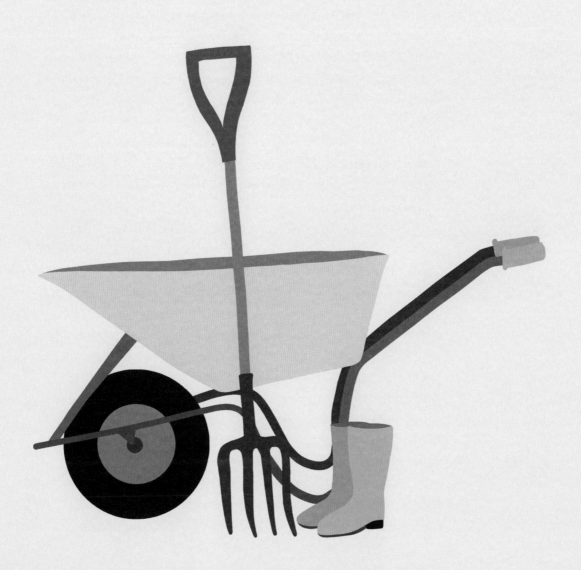

Get Creative with New Life
Getting started with seeds and cuttings

There is a reason why TV gardening shows constantly cover the subject of sowing seeds or creating new plants from cuttings. It is absolutely fascinating. We are mesmerized by new life, and this is the epitome of it. We cut a small piece of stem from a shoot (known as a softwood cutting) on a parent plant, place it in a glass of water or a pot of free-draining growing medium (compost), and voilà, we have a whole plant with lovely new roots just three weeks later! Even after 50 years of gardening, I am still astounded by the capacity of this little piece of green stem to generate new cells and morph into a whole new plant.

Seeds are just as captivating: a whole plant tucked away in a tiny nutshell (quite literally) and held in suspended animation. Seed cells survive in a dehydrated state and have their own 'larder' of food (the endosperm) to keep them ticking over, waiting for nature (or us) to provide the right triggers. They are ready for the long haul – perhaps one winter season, or perhaps ten, before germination will take place. Seeds are nature's equivalent of the long-distance space capsule, with all the requirements for life packaged in a tiny compartment.

Growing plants from seed is great fun and a distraction from the routines of modern life. There is something special about nurturing a young living entity, investing time and effort into the encouragement of this new life. The key is placing the growing seeds somewhere that is suitable for them, but also for you. A windowsill that you pass frequently – perhaps in the kitchen or bathroom – is ideal, somewhere you can keep an eye on your progeny.

Different plants have different requirements, so it's important to follow the instructions closely if you have bought a packet of seeds.

Many require a specific temperature, and the growing medium should be kept moist, but not waterlogged. Some require light, while others shun it until they have germinated. A useful gardener's trick for seeds that you are unsure about is to place a sheet of newspaper over the seed tray or pot. This will block out enough light for those species that prefer the dark, but allow through enough for those that require light to germinate.

Creating young plants from cuttings is considered a green art, but it is very much a science, too. Most things want to live; it is just a matter of putting them in the right environmental conditions to foster this inherent drive for survival. Biologically speaking, cuttings fall into two camps. The first is those with pre-formed root cells embedded in the stems, and it is just a matter of coaxing these out, usually by putting them in water or a damp growing medium.

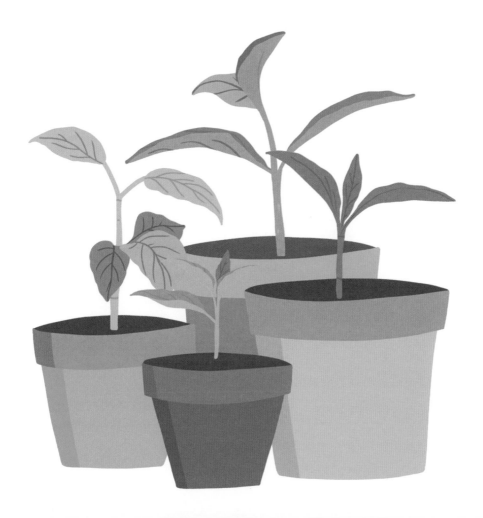

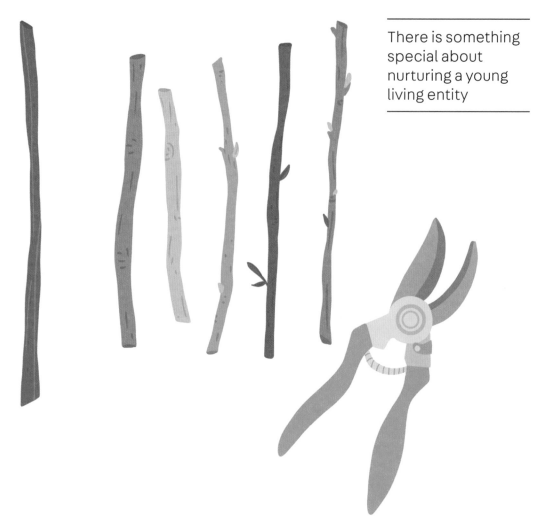

Jargon-buster

Cuttings actually come in four types, not just softwood cuttings. Semi-hardwood cuttings are similar to softwood cuttings but stiffer, in that part of the stem has begun to form lignin (wood). Hardwood cuttings are formed from 'hard', fully lignified stems (the stronger stems that allow woody plants to form a skeletal structure that stands up against gravity and, indeed, withstands many a storm). This type is conventionally rooted over winter by placing the woody stems in the ground and leaving them undisturbed until spring. Such plants as dogwood (*Cornus*), currants (*Ribes*) and shrub roses (for example, *Rosa mundi*) are propagated in this way.

The final type of cutting is a root cutting, where everything is in reverse. Dig up a piece of root, chop it into small sections and lay it just below the surface of the growing medium. Keep it moist and in a few weeks shoots will start to appear. New baby plants from old roots! Oriental poppies (*Papaver orientale*) and the stunning paper-petalled tree poppy, *Romneya coulteri*, among other things, are propagated using this method.

Plants such as willow (*Salix*), poplar (*Populus*), *Fuchsia* and tomato (*Lycopersicon esculentum*) fall into this category.

The second group need to generate new roots, after a wound response (triggered by us taking the cutting) induces the formation of undifferentiated cells. These cells have the potential to form any part of the plant (stem, leaf, flower or root), but they are prompted to form new roots by the environment in which they find themselves, in this case moist growing medium. (Confusingly, in medical circles, cells that have the potential to form any type of organ are called 'stem' cells, but medical doctors are not thinking about green shoots when they refer to them.)

Success with cuttings is all about keeping them hydrated until they can form their own roots and become self-sufficient in terms of water. So they must be kept out of direct sunlight, but still have access to enough light for them to make sugars through photosynthesis. High humidity helps, too – so that north-facing bathroom windowsill (south-facing in the southern hemisphere) will come in handy. Alternatively, cover the pots of cuttings with a clear polythene bag to keep humidity high.

Most plants root within three weeks, but some may take a lot longer. In general, ease of rooting is inversely related to the stature of the plant. Short, soft-stemmed bedding and herbaceous plants are easiest to root, then woody shrubs; trees are the most challenging (with some exceptions; see willow and poplar above). In fact, trees are often grafted (which involves making a physical union of two different species – a rootstock and a scion) because of the difficulty or slowness of generating new plants from cuttings.

Doze by a Bubble Stone

2 | **De-stress by listening to the sound of running water**

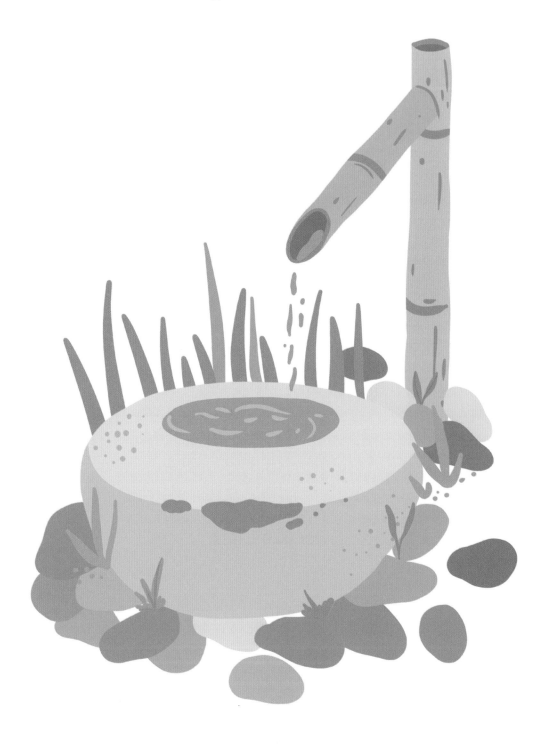

People are attracted to water in different ways. Views of water are frequently considered attractive or mesmerizing. Water is associated with a change in the atmosphere, and we sense the higher humidity associated with a river or lake, or smell the salt on the wind when we are close to the sea. We also recognize that the landscape changes near water, as does the type and diversity of wildlife.

Our hunter-gatherer ancestors realized that ponds and rivers were important places for finding food as well as water. Seascapes and coastal features supplied novel and readily attainable food sources (such as shellfish) and were ideal for gaining vantage points. They were also the superhighways of their day and, unlike the impenetrable forests that covered most of the land, allowed relative ease of movement. Small family groups would move along the coast or up river valleys, stopping from time to time to interact with each other. Some psychologists believe that this is why we are hardwired to search out water in the landscape today.

Important aspects in the sensual perception of water are its sound, colour, clarity, motion and context. People are entranced by the sound of water, and we attach great importance to the variety and special nature of those sounds, from calm ripples to an energetic roar. Both the calming sound and the visual movement of running water are restorative.

Not everyone can see the ocean from their garden, but almost anyone can enjoy the relaxing sound of moving water by creating a small water feature. An almost limitless range of products is available from garden centres and online, including:

- the classic pond with a fountain in the middle
- a 'natural' mini-waterfall tumbling over three or four strata of rock
- bespoke products, such as a pebble pool, a statue or a stone ball with built-in bubble fountain
- a rocky 'plunge' pool with water overflowing from an amphora

- a mock wishing well with leaky collecting bucket that trickles water back down the well

Any water feature with a pump must have a safe external source of electricity. Many are powered by solar panels and can be easily installed by the layperson; otherwise, consult a qualified electrician.

If you have a garden with a decent slope, you could even create your own mountain stream or babbling brook. Simply run a hidden hose from a water pump immersed in a receiver pond up to a high point and conceal it within a carefully created rocky outcrop or scree. Make a stream bed by laying a waterproof butyl or plastic liner down to the pond, keeping it in place with rocks or boulders and backfilling the 'stream bed' with an aggregate of your choice. For a modernist feel and added colour, choose ground-down, smooth coloured glass as a recycled aggregate material. More traditionally, water running over a slate cascade or between granite pebbles is magical, both visually – in the way the water flows and contorts its way down the stream bed – and aurally, from the trickling and gurgling sounds that result. Close your eyes and you will be transported to a Welsh mountain valley or a lost gorge in the Himalayas.

For those who do not have a natural slope, a more obviously human-orientated water feature is more desirable. A waterspout emerging from a wall or a tap (faucet) linked to an old water trough will look less incongruous than a stream that is artificially hoisted above a flat landscape.

Plants by water

Consider reinforcing your escapist world with astute plantings by your water feature.

For the Welsh valley theme, consider allowing the sulphur-coloured Welsh poppy (*Papaver cambricum*) to self-seed among the slate chips, and try one or two shuttlecock ferns (*Matteuccia struthiopteris*) beside the stream to give that dank feel. Over time, moss will naturally colonize the wet zone around the cascade.

For your Himalayan ideal, plant your choice of Asiatic primulas (such as *Primula pulverulenta*, *P. japonica*, *P. bulleyana*, *P. beesiana*, *P. florindae* and *P. vialii*, which cover an array of pinks, reds, yellows, oranges and purples) to brighten the streamside in early summer. You may also wish to embroider the pebble 'beaches' with smaller-leaved *Hosta* cultivars, their rounded leaves matching the form of the stones. You can even have something to look at in winter by planting a low-growing *Rhododendron* or *Pieris* on the upper part of the scree.

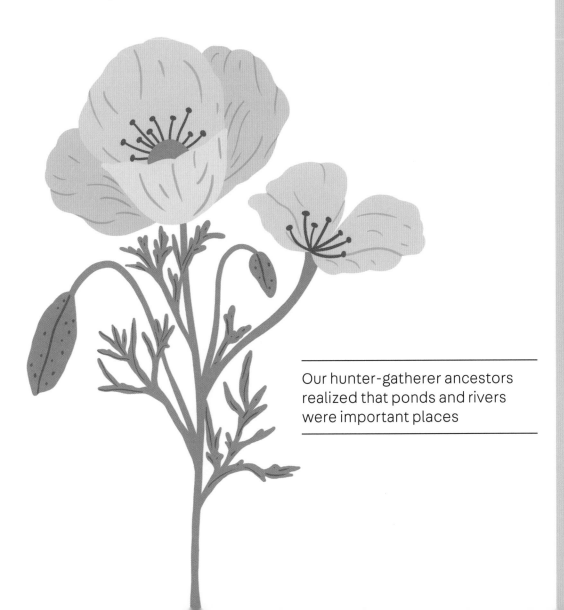

Our hunter-gatherer ancestors realized that ponds and rivers were important places

Play with Jurassic Plants
Create an otherworldly feel with cycads and ferns

3

There is nothing quite like getting away from it all. So how about stepping millions of years back in time to the era of the dinosaurs? I don't mean literally, of course, but rather by tapping into that most powerful of organs: the human brain. Humans have an astonishing capacity to imagine what the past was like. Indeed, we can use our memory and learned experience to re-create other worlds, in terms of both time and place. What's more, these imaginary processes are likely to be therapeutic. According to the Attention Restoration theory (see pages 9 and 122–3), being away from the source of our directed attention (mental tasks that require concentration and that add to our stress) is important. The good thing is that we can remove ourselves 'virtually' from these intensive mental tasks to gain the benefits; we do not need to move physically away. So don't underrate the importance of the imagination, which can be a catalyst for escapism and let us forget the source of our stress.

Many people are entranced by a particular garden style, whether a wild garden, jungle garden, desert garden, Edwardian flower garden, cottage garden, formal country-house garden or any other type. But there is also the option to explore prehistory by creating, for example, a primeval Jurassic-era garden. Plants first evolved about 870 million years ago, and by the Jurassic (200 million years ago) the planet was covered with forests of conifers, such as monkey puzzle (*Araucaria araucana*) and dawn redwood (*Metasequoia glyptostroboides*). Also present were other gymnosperms (plants with naked, not enclosed, seeds), such as maidenhair trees (*Ginkgo biloba*), podocarps (a type of conifer) and cycads (palm-like species). There were forests of tree ferns, and the forest floor would have been dominated by mosses, horsetails and other ferns. Flowering plants, and their friends the bees, had not yet arrived on the scene.

Make a bold impression with one or two plants

Your Jurassic garden should be dominated by bold green forms; this is the land of the dinosaur, after all. You don't need lots of space, but you do want to make a bold impression with one or two plants, and create the notion of being on the fringes of a deeper primeval forest. The boldness could come from a cycad, with large fronds arching in lovely symmetrical curves. Cycads are not fully winter-hardy, but an alternative is the sago palm (*Cycas revoluta*), which can stay outdoors all year round in milder locations; in regions where temperatures dip below -5°C (23°F) it is best kept in a container and moved to a bright spot indoors in winter.

I would give pride of place to *Metasequoia glyptostroboides.* This is a genuine fossil tree, being known only from fossil records until a small population was discovered in central China in 1941. The species itself can grow big, but the lovely gold-needle cultivars, such as 'Gold Rush' and 'Amber Glow', are less vigorous and can be kept in check with judicial annual pruning. *Ginkgo biloba*, with its olive-green 'duck-foot' leaves, can likewise be kept tame with an annual shear. Don't forget to fill the gaps at ground level with ferns. *Dryopteris wallichiana* will throw up fronds that mimic the relaxed curves of the cycad. *Asplenium scolopendrium*, the hart's-tongue fern, with its bolder, more substantial leaves, provides a useful contrast. There won't be room for an actual dinosaur, I suspect, but you could replace one of the patio pavers with a home-cast footprint of a predatory *Ceratosaurus*.

Health Benefit
Air Quality

People often say 'Step outside and get some fresh air', implying the health-promoting and refreshing nature of being outdoors. But is our air really that fresh? Sadly, these days, that notion is being challenged, at least for those who live in a town or city. Air quality is a big problem in most cities across the globe, and can be attributed largely to emissions from vehicles, factories, coal-fired power stations and, particularly in the developing world, the burning of charcoal, wood and animal dung for cooking. Poor-quality air accounts for 6.67 million deaths worldwide each year, and, heart-breakingly, for the premature death of some 500,000 babies annually. Even in countries with some form of emissions regulations, premature death is attributed to polluted atmospheres; in the European Union, for example, it accounts for 630,000 additional deaths every year.

Pollutants in the air include gaseous elements, such as nitrous and sulphur oxides, carbon monoxide, ozone and volatile organic compounds (VOCs). By-products of combustion also cause problems, and the 'smuts' and 'soots' form particulate matter that is categorized by size (PM_{10}, $PM_{2.5}$ and PM_1). These soot particles can also contain heavy-metal molecules, such as lead. Not only do pollutants damage our lungs directly and cause subsequent respiratory problems, but also the smaller particles and molecules are absorbed directly into the bloodstream, leading to cardiovascular disease and other chronic problems.

The answer to poor-quality air is to reduce emissions, but where this is not possible, plants can partially mitigate effects at a local level. They work particularly well when used as a barrier between the source of pollution, for example a road, and the people who are affected by it. Plants reduce pollutant loads in the air by filtering out the pollutants, adhering some of the particles to their leaves, and absorbing and/or biologically deactivating some of the compounds.

The effectiveness of plants in trapping and deactivating aerial pollutants depends on the species, the design with respect to the main source of pollution (since poor design can make air quality worse), and the density or complexity of the planting. Wider vegetation barriers and those comprising plants of varying height and density work best. Plants that have a large surface area (many small, closely spaced leaves, for example), or leaf shapes or properties that help to trap particles, are especially beneficial.[1] In this sense, leaves that have many folds or hairs, or a rough or sticky (waxy) surface, tend to trap more particles than those with smooth or non-waxy leaves.

Air pollution is no joke, and plants can help only so far. Ultimately, we must get to the root of the problem and move to cleaner sources of energy.

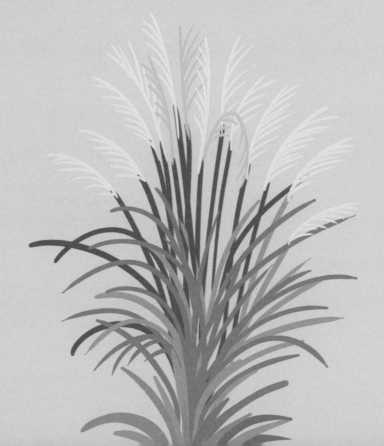

Breathe in the Fresh Air
Plants that stop 'sick building syndrome'

4

'Sick building syndrome' is a misnomer, since it is really the residents who are sick, not the building. It is the name for a phenomenon whereby people in buildings – usually office blocks – suffer from nasal irritation, dry throat, sore eyes, headache and nausea. The precise cause is unclear, but such symptoms are often aligned with buildings that have poor natural ventilation or problems with heating and air-conditioning units. Even in our own homes, we can find that the rooms are excessively dry or stuffy. Opening a window can be one of the first remedies, but modern commercial buildings may not have openable windows. And, if you live next to a major road, for example, opening a window may actually reduce air quality as well as increase noise.

Whether in the office or at home, you might find that your interior environment is improved by the addition of a few houseplants. Plants raise the local humidity through transpiration, which is to say that they release water vapour from the undersides of their leaves as they photosynthesize. Ideally, building interiors should have between 40 and 70 per cent relative humidity, and plants with large leaves and strong transpiration rates – such as the heartleaf philodendron (*Philodendron hederaceum*) or the Swiss cheese plant (*Monstera deliciosa*) – can help to maintain this level. They also look fantastic. My Swiss cheese plant has been with me for 27 years and currently sprawls across the bedroom windowsill, its serrated leaves judiciously guarding the wardrobe door. For larger houseplants such as these, it is useful to place the pot in a shallow tray that you keep topped up with water. This reduces the amount of water splash on your furniture, and provides a shallow pool that itself raises humidity. This benefits the plant as well as the human occupants of the room.

The other common contributors to poor indoor air quality are the volatile organic compounds or VOCs. These are small organic molecules that vaporize readily into the air and thus equally readily enter our respiratory systems. You may be familiar with some, such as acetone, trichloroethylene, formaldehyde and benzene, and these and similar compounds are released from everyday objects such as printers, carpets, paints and cleaning products. Plants capture and deactivate these compounds, both directly (such as through their leaves) and indirectly, by supporting beneficial microbial communities that occur on their leaves and roots. ('Phylloplane' and 'rhizosphere' microbiota, respectively, since you ask.)

The idea of plants 'scrubbing' the air was first researched by the American space agency NASA. It was looking for plants to improve the air quality on spacecraft for astronauts undertaking long journeys in confined conditions, but householders and office workers have benefited from its findings. A lovely display of peace lily (*Spathiphyllum wallisii*), sword fern (*Nephrolepis exaltata*), mother-in-law's tongue (*Sansevieria trifasciata*) and Asian royal fern (*Osmunda japonica*) could be used to adorn a workspace. If there is room on the floor, try a rubber plant (*Ficus elastica*) in an ornamental container. If you want bona fide species initially evaluated for NASA, you might add a spider plant (*Chlorophytum comosum*) or golden pothos (*Scindapsus aureus*).

5 Try a Yogurt Tree
Grow a lemon tree in a reused pot

Fruit is designed for our pleasure. That's why it is sweet like the strawberry, tangy like the tomato, or even slightly bitter as in the lemon (or, as we would say in my home country of Scotland, wersh) – to stimulate the taste buds. For millennia plants have been conning us to taste their fruit, eat their seeds and thus distribute their progeny across the countryside, to help them establish new colonies. Even today, you might notice the occasional apple tree by the side of a road or footpath. Nobody planted that tree deliberately, but someone threw away an apple core in that spot several decades back. We are not the only ones conned; birds, monkeys and fruit-eating bats are too.

Creating new life from plant parts is a great activity (see chapter 1), but it is even better when you can do it from unusual sources, such as those fruit peelings you are about to put in the bin. It is gratifying to create a whole new tree from something you would normally discard, and it's a great way to teach children about the cycle of life.

For a lemon tree, the recipe for new life is:

• Take one organic, unwaxed lemon bought from the grocer or supermarket.
• Use the lemon in the normal way – as zest in a cake, perhaps, or as slices in drinks – and retain the seeds.
• Suck the seeds for a few moments (this may look strange to other occupants of the kitchen), rinse them in tap water for 4–5 minutes, or leave them soaking overnight in a dish of water. This will remove any clinging flesh and, more importantly, wash off any natural chemical inhibitors to germination. These inhibitors stop seeds from germinating too early or in the wrong place;

it's not the brightest idea for the lemon to germinate inside the fruit itself, or in your stomach, for that matter. Normally these inhibitors are removed as the seed goes through the gut or experiences some other 'weathering' process.

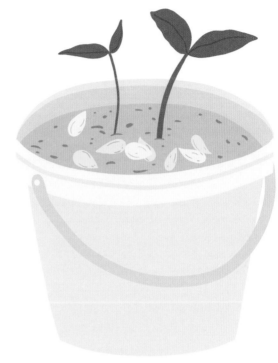

- Dry the seeds carefully using paper towels.
- Take a clean yogurt pot and pierce five or six holes in the base. (The pot must be scrupulously clean; prolific fungal growth is not the aim of this exercise, and it could be detrimental to the young seedling.)
- Fill the pot with a proprietary growing medium for seedlings, avoiding unsustainably harvested peat.
- Place the seeds on the growing medium and press them in gently about 2cm (¾in), so that they are covered.
- Cover the pot with clear polythene and place it on a saucer on a bright windowsill (but not in direct sunlight) at 15–22°C (60–72°F).
- Wait patiently for 3–6 weeks for the new green shoots to appear. The time it takes for the seeds to germinate will depend on how much of the inhibitor you removed.

Make sure you buy a lemon that actually has fully formed seed inside. Organically grown fruit are more likely to have viable seed, because conventional commercial growers can trick plants into forming fruit without pollination taking place. These are called parthenocarpic fruit. The process is used when it is too cold for pollinating insects to be active, for example, or where it is not desirable to have seed in the fruit – as with seedless grapes.

Be aware that what you get from your new tree will not be what you had in the fruit. A seed from a Meyer lemon may have only half

The need to chill out

Many of the trees that are native to temperate regions produce seed that needs a period of cold before it can break dormancy and germinate. This exposure to cold is called stratification. Apples, cherries, pears and peaches fall into this category. The process for germinating these seeds is the same as for the lemon, except that, rather than sowing the seed fresh from the fruit, place them in the refrigerator for two or three months. Layer them in damp paper towels, fold them into a polythene bag, then place at the back of the refrigerator (not in the freezer). Put a sticky note on the fridge door to make sure you don't forget about them.

the genes of the mother plant, since the pollen may have come from another type of lemon growing nearby. Each seed has two parents, but the fruit itself has only one, the flesh being composed of tissue from the mother plant alone. This is one reason why many fruit trees are produced by grafting (fusing a bud of the desired cultivar on to a rootstock of a different genetic make-up, thus producing a clone).

In any case, the lemon tree you produce will be your own unique product. Depending on where you live, you can keep it indoors, plant it out (in the mildest climates) or keep it inside in winter and place it on a warm patio in summer. Lemon trees produce lovely glossy green leaves, white citrus-scented flowers and citrus-yellow, lime-green or sometimes pink-flushed fruit that is ideal for making your own lemonade. More importantly, lemons are a rich source of vitamin C.

> Creating new life
> from plant parts
> is a great activity

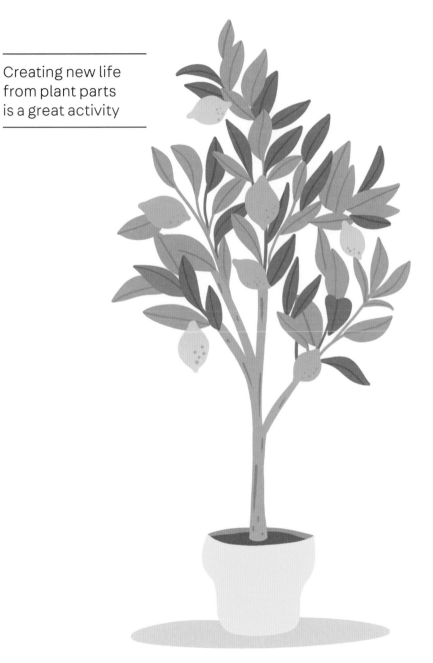

Vitamin C

Fruit – lemons in particular – is full of vitamin C (ascorbic acid). This is essential for human metabolic reactions, including extracting energy from food, and for improving immunity. It's therefore no surprise that many cold and flu remedies are flavoured with lemon. Vitamin C also aids the absorption of iron, another key component in our immunity. The role of vitamin C is wider than this, though; it helps to synthesize collagen, which is important for connective tissues and for speeding up recovery from wounds.

Mediterranean Vitality

6 Grow Mediterranean herbs in your window box

The Mediterranean diet is a very healthy one, and the generous use of herbs contributes to this. Mediterranean culinary herbs produce a range of chemicals that are known as phytoncides (or, more simply, essential oils) because the plant uses them to keep pests and pathogens away, and to make its leaves unpalatable to grazing animals. This is important for plants that grow in an environment that is too arid to allow them to make new leaves quickly. One of the 'design faults' of this strategy, though, is that these compounds are attractive to humans, and we exploit them to spice up our food. (Evolutionarily speaking, it is not a fault at all, of course, as these species now grow across the globe – a definite sign of success in the plant world.)

Herbs not only improve the aroma and flavour of our staple foods, but also protect us from acute disease. Their leaves contain antioxidants, which protect our cells from free radicals, those wayward ions that damage membranes and other parts of our cells. The leaves are full of alkaloids, phenolic diterpenes, flavonoids and polyphenols, substances that work together to inhibit inflammatory responses and to avoid the malfunction of cells and the formation of tumours. As if that were not enough, these compounds aid brain activity, regulate mood and lower cholesterol. They are super-compounds indeed.

Humans often find these aromas attractive and soothing, hence their use in aromatherapy. Dieticians originally assumed that we had to eat these herbs in order to get the physical benefits, but even just breathing in the aroma (the volatile oils) may be beneficial (see pages 172–3).

Parsley, sage, rosemary and thyme

Or so the song goes. Actually, since the boffin botanists have recently reclassified rosemary as a type of sage (it was originally *Rosmarinus* but is now *Salvia*), the lyrics in any new cover versions should be the rather less catchy 'Parsley, sage, sage and thyme'. Irrespective of the subtleties of plant nomenclature and musical taste, how about a window box of herbs near the kitchen so that you have ready access to fresh leaves when cooking? You might consider oregano (*Origanum vulgare*), parsley (*Petroselinum crispum*) and dill (*Anethum graveolens*). Alternatively, you could site pots of basil (*Ocimum basilicum*), sage (*Salvia officinalis*), rosemary (*Salvia rosmarinus*) and lavender (*Lavandula angustifolia*) near the back door. Depending on your olfactory sensitivity, it might be prudent to place the pungent garlic (*Allium sativum*) and clove (*Syzygium aromaticum*) a bit further away. Finally, furnish your garden paths with thyme (*Thymus*). Allow the mat- and carpet-forming types (such as *T. vulgaris*, *T. 'Dartmoor'* and *T. serpyllum* 'Petite') to grow in the joints between paving stones, and edge the paths with taller varieties, such as *T. citriodorus* 'Variegatus', *T. pulegioides* 'Bertram Anderson' and *T. serpyllum* 'Elfin'.

Herbs not only improve the aroma and flavour of our staple foods, but also protect us from acute disease

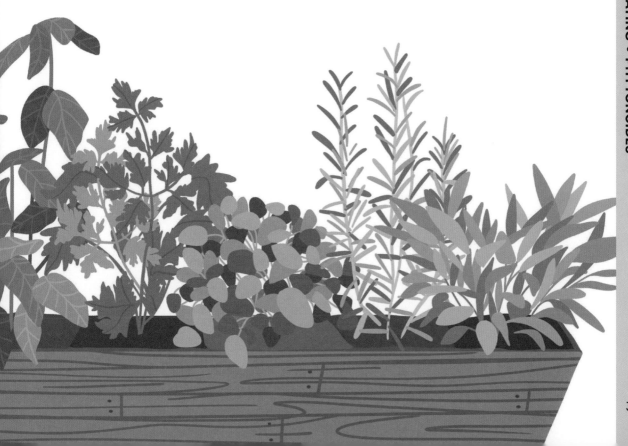

7 | Watch the Mini-bugs
Create a pond or mini-meadow for a world of insects

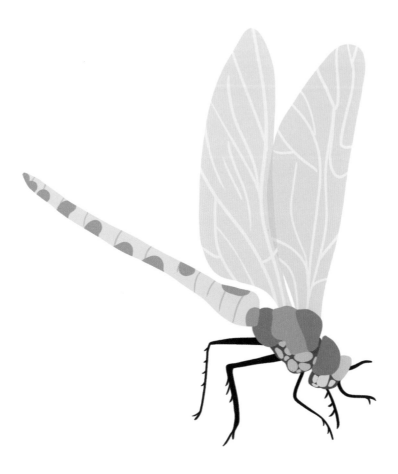

Engaging with plants and gardening should be about taking a broader, more fundamental step closer to the natural world. I am attracted to the beauty of my garden plants, but I also see them as habitat for other life. If I can strike a balance between maintaining the health and aesthetics of my plants and helping wildlife, I am a happy gardener. For example, I really don't mind greenfly (aphids) on my roses. They normally don't affect the flowers, and I know that if I don't have aphids, I don't have hoverflies and blue tits (or chickadees in North America), and if I don't have those, I certainly won't have swallows or sparrowhawks. My garden is part of nature's food chain, not a sterile pleasure dome. If I notice that the aphids are reaching plague proportions on a plant, I can always rub them off with my fingers – not revert to pesticides. If you can develop a well-balanced garden with effective ecological links, you rarely need to take drastic action.

By adopting this nonchalant attitude, you will actually start to appreciate the little crawly, burrowing and buzzy critters that call your garden home. Flowering plants provide colour and wonder, but so do red admiral butterflies, broad-bodied chaser dragonflies (the males have a powder-blue body and the females are golden-ochre) and buff-tailed bumblebees in their striped rugby shirts. North American dragonflies include the eastern pondhawk, with powder-blue males and emerald-green females with black-and-white stripes. These creatures are not just ornamental; observe them carefully to uncover a fascinating world of subtle interaction and high drama.

It's an old adage that if you want life in the garden, add a pond. And if you do, my goodness does life come in quickly. Every time I have constructed a pond, within about three days pond-skaters (pond striders) have come to check it out. Although these insects don't look like the archetypal flying machines, with their narrow, 'two-dimensional' bodies and splayed legs, they are obviously adept at air travel, at spotting new ponds and new opportunities. Such surface surfers are on the hunt for small midges and gnats that get stuck in the surface tension of the water. They have sensitive hairs on their legs that allow them to pick up the smallest vibration on the surface of the pond and home in on their prey.

The next colonizers are the single-cell algae that form phytoplankton in the warm upper parts of the pond, often turning the water a deep pea-green. The 'munchers' soon get to work on that and the small animals that constitute the zooplankton begin to take a toll on the microscopic plants, but be aware that the water in a natural pond will never be completely clear again.

With time, a fully functioning network of life will become apparent. No two ponds will be identical, since factors such as water pH, sunlight and nutrient levels will determine what plants and animals are present and in what proportions. Typical stars of the show are the 'predatory dragons', dragonfly and damselfly nymphs. Some of the mature nymphs of the larger species are quite capable of impaling a small fish or tadpole with their extendable mouthparts.

Invest in a good guidebook and enjoy identifying the tiny but amazing life forms in your pond. Keep an eye out for the 'battle-hardened shields' (actually the elytra, or protective wing covers) of the great diving beetle and various common diving beetles (water tigers in North America) as they commute from the bottom of the pond to the surface to breathe. More animated are the whirligig beetles (including the appropriately named *Gyrinus substriatus*), which gyrate on the surface of the water. Handily, they have two pairs of compound eyes: one pair for seeing below and the other for viewing above the surface. The little guys that look like submerged sculling boats are called water boatmen, and are a predatory bug. They will scarper to the bottom when your shadow crosses the pond.

Mini-meadows are a super way to bring pollinating insects and other invertebrates into your garden. Annual 'meadows' of poppies (*Papaver rhoeas*), cornflowers (*Centaurea cyanus*), corn marigolds (*Glebionis segetum*) and so on are very colourful and provide pollen and nectar for a wide range of pollinating species. Generally, you must sow these plant communities every winter in cultivated soil, unless your garden is on free-draining sandy soil, where they can perpetuate themselves through self-seeding from one year to the next. Just remove the dead plants in midwinter and hoe over the ground in late winter or early spring to remove any perennial weeds.

Flower-filled annual meadows are useful for drawing in some of the key pollinator groups, such as butterflies, bees and hoverflies, while true meadows – which are actually composed of grasses and broad-leaved perennial plants (known as forbs) – bring in a wider range of insects, including grasshoppers, true bugs and beetles such as ladybirds (ladybugs) and predatory ground beetles. Quite a number of butterfly species depend on meadow grass as food for their caterpillars, giving further justification for small areas of perennial meadow. The key to a perennial meadow is to let the forbs flower and form viable seeds, then cut all the vegetation back to about 10cm (4in) in late summer.

Don't expect an instant mass of flower colour, though; true meadows are ecological laboratories in which plants jostle for success and dominance, but they are at the mercy of the wider environment. What you see in a dry year may be very different from a subsequent wet year. To avoid the more vigorous grasses and forbs dominating, consider adding the hemi-parasitic plant yellow rattle (*Rhinanthus minor*). It can bring some of the stronger-growing 'thugs' to their knees by tapping into their roots and stealing their sugars, thus levelling the playing field for other species. It is an annual, so make sure you create some small bare patches over winter (a good pull of a rake through the meadow will do the job) to give its seeds space to germinate in the spring. In North America Canadian lousewort (*Pedicularis canadensis*) does a similar job in keeping the more vigorous prairie grasses in check.

It's an old adage that if you want life in the garden, add a pond

Orchid Opulence
Cultivate orchids indoors

I can't move in our house for orchids. They inhabit every room, and there are even two in the bath. The house looks like a DIY store just before Christmas, when the orchids are 'packed high' for sale. I can take no credit for these lovely plants; they are all my partner's doing. You don't need much imagination in the face of this level of restorative greenery to feel immersed in a relaxing tropical paradise.

When in flower, these exotic beauties transform any room. We have a moth orchid, *Phalaenopsis* 'Kung's Green Star', with enormous blooms of the palest green, performing in the bedroom. *P. grandiflorum* 'Rio Grande' dominates the spare room with its exquisite cerise-pink flower, and one of the bath-blockers is *P.* 'Elegant Polka Dots', white with broad pink spots. There is a *Cymbidium* 'Loch Lomond' (lemon flowers with red ringing the lowest petal, known as the lip) in the living room; this one is moved to a semi-shady place outdoors in summer because it needs good indirect sunlight to form its flowers.

Most orchids you see for sale are *Phalaenopsis*, and surprisingly easy to care for. These are epiphytes, the plant equivalent of the sloth, which is to say that in nature they spend all their life hanging off trees in tropical rainforests. This gives clues about how to look after them. They live below the canopies of great trees, so they want filtered, not direct, sunlight. High humidity but not soggy conditions keeps them happy, since their roots normally hang in free air or explore decaying leaf litter in the boughs of a tree. You will notice that orchids are sold in translucent pots to let light reach the roots. This is because the roots also photosynthesize, so keep them in this type of pot when potting on. Put these elements together and a bathroom location out of direct sunlight sounds about right.

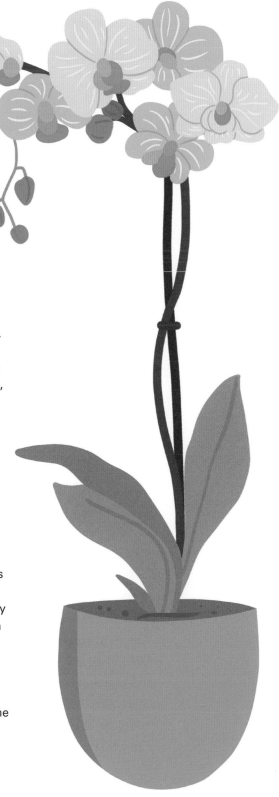

Orchids are the most diverse plant family on Earth

Orchids: Biodiversity of their own

The variety of colours, shapes and sizes among orchid flowers is immense. This is the most diverse plant family on Earth, with more than 30,000 species. Some are found only in tiny, isolated populations in the wild. Orchids hybridize easily across species, throwing up lots of cultivated forms for the houseplant trade. It is this diversity and rarity, along with their beauty, that have made orchids famous.

This is also why some people become so immersed in them. Orchids allow one to delve into a hobby and be transfixed by the enormous variety. Such total absorption is an ideal distraction from work and the other stresses and strains of everyday life. It is a good thing, as long as it is not taken to excess (see chapter 37), and this is true both for us humans and for the orchids. The orchid family has been decimated by over-collection from the wild and exploitation driven by demand from amateur growers, who wish to possess something rare. Thankfully, most orchids on the market now are raised en masse through micropropagation, although there is still some illegal trading of wild plants. If in any doubt, buy only varieties with cultivar names.

9

Cultivate the Fruit of the Andes
Grow tomatoes on your windowsill

The tomato is an enigma. It is actually a fruit, but is treated as a vegetable because of its savoury taste. Its alternative name is 'love apple', but no one is sure if that has to do with its supposedly aphrodisiac properties, or with a grammatical mix-up during the sixteenth century. The plant was discovered in Central America and introduced to the Old World by the Spanish, but it entered Morocco via the Spanish Moors, and the Moroccans called it *mala oethiopica*, 'apple of the Moors'. The Italians then called it the same thing, *pomi dei mori*, which the French misinterpreted as *pommes d'amour*, 'apples of love', and the English translated to 'love apples'. To add to the confusion, the scientific name, *Lycopersicon esculentum*, translates as 'edible wolf peach' – not an apple in sight. The conflicting theme continues when we find that the 'love apple' is also associated with Aztec cannibalism (tomatoes being the moderating side dish, presumably), and that, although the fruit is edible, the rest of the plant is poisonous. It was thus rightly distrusted by Europeans when first imported.

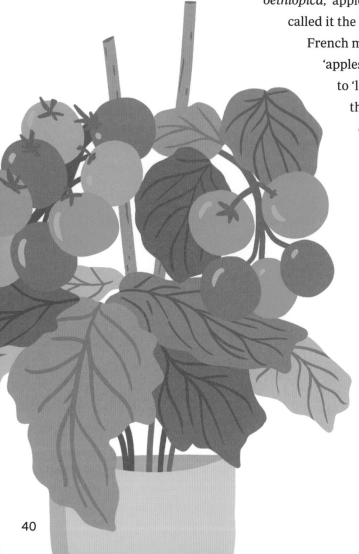

The tomato is a useful part of our diet thanks to a range of health-promoting properties

Despite its turbulent ethnobotany, the tomato is a useful part of our diet thanks to a range of health-promoting properties. Tomatoes contain lycopene, which is noted both for its anti-cancer properties and for its capacity to counteract cardiovascular disease. They provide fibre, potassium and vitamins A, B, C, E and K (the last of which is important for blood clotting and wound healing). They are also linked to providing protection against macular degeneration, as well as alleviating symptoms of the menopause. Middle-aged women who drank tomato juice for eight weeks had fewer menopausal symptoms and lower anxiety, were more physically active, and had a stronger heart rate and lower triglyceride levels (high triglycerides are linked to heart disease) than those who did not.[2] Unlike other vegetables, which are best eaten fresh, tomatoes seem to have greater benefits when cooked, since cooking enhances antioxidant activity and lycopene levels.

Not just tomato-red

We think of tomatoes as red, but in fact the original plants brought to Europe probably had golden fruit. Their colour varies markedly today, with varieties in green ('Green Envy'), creamy-yellow ('Cream Sausage'), lemon-yellow ('Limoncito'), orange ('Sungold'), plum ('Rosella') and almost black ('Black Opal'), and some that are tiger-striped ('Tiger Red') or mottled ('Midnight Snack'). Add to this the great variety of shapes and you will quickly realize that the old love apple is ornamental as well as delicious.

In warm climates, tomatoes can be grown outdoors, but in more temperate areas you may want to use a greenhouse or sunny windowsill. Start with the cherry and other small types of tomato, because they ripen more readily than the larger types. There are dwarf or patio varieties, which are ideal for small spaces and do not require the tying-in that the taller, heavier varieties demand. Cultivars such as 'Totem', 'Balconi', 'Vilma', 'Rosella Crimson' and 'Sweet 'n' Neat' are either compact or trailing, and fit easily into a window space. With time you might try some of the conventional 'bush' types. Beware, though: as a teenager I tied some 'Ailsa Craig' tomato plants to strings attached to the curtain rail in my bedroom. By the end of the summer I had a reasonable crop of tomatoes but also a U-shaped curtain rail. It wasn't my most popular period with my parents.

Health Benefit
Noise Reduction

Noise is not only annoying; it can also be a killer. Persistent or loud environmental noise, such as that from road traffic or aircraft, negatively affects sleep quality and cardiovascular health. The World Health Organization estimates that the number of 'years of quality life' lost in EU states through noise pollution is 61,000 (via heart disease) and 903,000 (via sleep disturbance). Different people experience noise in different ways. Some suffer 'noise annoyance', becoming more anxious. This means that noise can

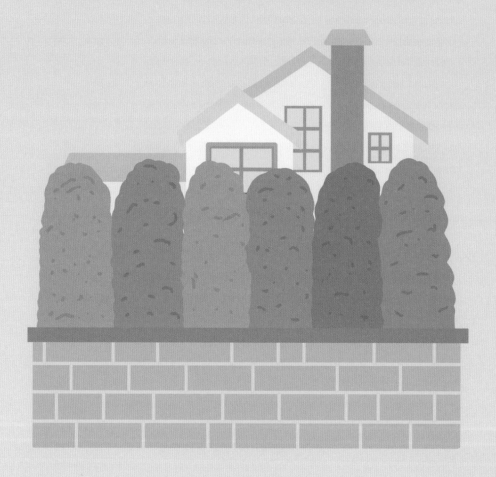

interfere with daily activities, feelings, thoughts, rest or sleep, and it may be accompanied by emotional responses, such as irritability, exhaustion, distress and other stress-related symptoms. As well as being induced by predictable, consistent sound, noise annoyance can be brought on by unpredictable or infrequent sounds, such as barking dogs and noise from neighbours. It is thought to account for an additional 654,000 lost years of quality life.

Plants can help. A few plants won't stop a nearby noise completely, but they can reduce the volume by absorbing, reflecting, refracting and diffracting sound, as well as disrupting the sound wave patterns.[3] Essentially, plants have a muffling effect, and make noise less invasive and intrusive. The wider and thicker the planting you can put between you and the noise source, the better.

The amazing thing is that being in the presence of plants can make a location seem quieter even if it is not. The brain seems to register that when we enter a natural, well-planted environment it is 'mentally quieter', even though the decibels bombarding the ear have not changed. The perception of noise and the annoyance arising from it are not just physical, but also psychological. This is an important point to remember when we are designing our 'quiet', secluded sanctuaries.

Enjoy Peace and Quiet
Dampen intrusive noises using green barriers and facades

10

Urban living often correlates with a noisy existence, owing to the presence of cars, overhead aircraft, construction work and other industrial processes, and even the low-level hum of air-conditioning units. Many of us are exposed to constant noise, and even in our little havens of gardens or balconies, we can't guarantee that we can get away from it. The sounds of the city are all-pervasive, and over time they can be a cause of significant stress. But we can use plants to mitigate the effects. Different plants help against different noise wavelengths: fine-leaved species (such as *Cedrus deodara* and *Cryptomeria japonica*, both a type of cedar) deal with the low-frequency sound waves generated by traffic, whereas broader-leaved evergreens (such as *Photinia × fraseri* and the cherry laurel, *Prunus laurocerasus*) are better at absorbing high-frequency electrical noise.

Positioning plants correctly is important, of course. They must be between you and the source of the noise, which is not necessarily easy if a road runs parallel to your house. But placing plants in less obvious areas can also help. For example, growing climbers on the walls of your house stops incoming noise from rebounding or reverberating.

Sometimes engineers recommend solid walls and fences to block offending

Doubling up

When working from home, I will often head to the garden on sunny days, computer in hand. When the family is around, I find it quieter out there. We have designed our garden to have a 'double hedge' adjacent to a nearby field to help reduce noise from farm machinery. There is not a lot, but when it is harvest time it can be very disruptive. There is a 1m (3ft) gap between the two hedges and this seems to act as an extra 'insulator' to the external noise. The hedges themselves are a mix of species, including fine 'soft' and broad 'hard' leaf types, such as dogwood (*Cornus sanguinea*), field maple (*Acer campestre*), beech (*Fagus sylvatica*), white willow (*Salix alba* subsp. *vitellina* 'Willow Gold'), hornbeam (*Carpinus betulus*), privet (*Ligustrum ovalifolium*), shrubby honeysuckle (*Lonicera nitida*) and cherry laurel (*Prunus laurocerasus* 'Marbled White'), with wild dog rose (*Rosa canina*) for flower colour and guelder rose (*Viburnum opulus*) for its bright-red berries in autumn.

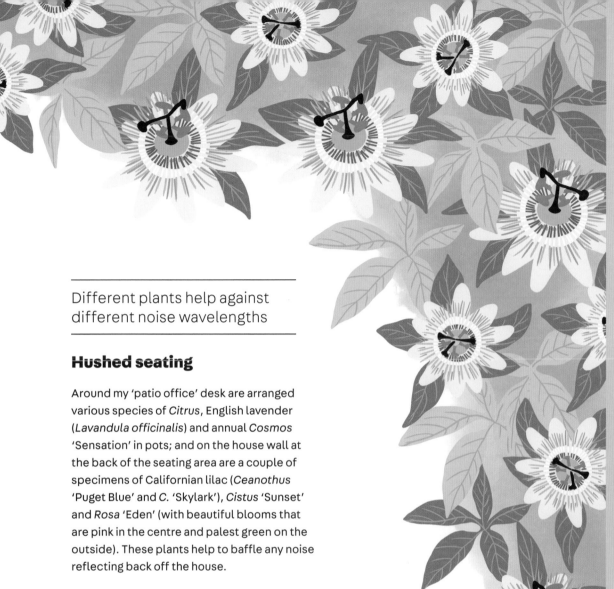

Different plants help against different noise wavelengths

Hushed seating

Around my 'patio office' desk are arranged various species of *Citrus*, English lavender (*Lavandula officinalis*) and annual *Cosmos* 'Sensation' in pots; and on the house wall at the back of the seating area are a couple of specimens of Californian lilac (*Ceanothus* 'Puget Blue' and *C.* 'Skylark'), *Cistus* 'Sunset' and *Rosa* 'Eden' (with beautiful blooms that are pink in the centre and palest green on the outside). These plants help to baffle any noise reflecting back off the house.

sounds, and these are effective. But covering them with climbers will increase the noise attenuation and look better, too. Wooden fences and brick walls are ideal for growing *Clematis*, and spectacular candy-striped cultivars, such as 'Doctor Ruppel', make a vibrant focal point.

Another approach is to swap annoying noise for more restful sounds. The gentle rustling of bamboo, for example, blocks human-derived noise, as does the 'positive' sound of a fountain or other water feature.

11

Natural Balance
Create a biodiversity 'hotspot'

The thrill of seeing a wild animal in the garden is difficult to describe, especially if it is a rare or unfamiliar creature

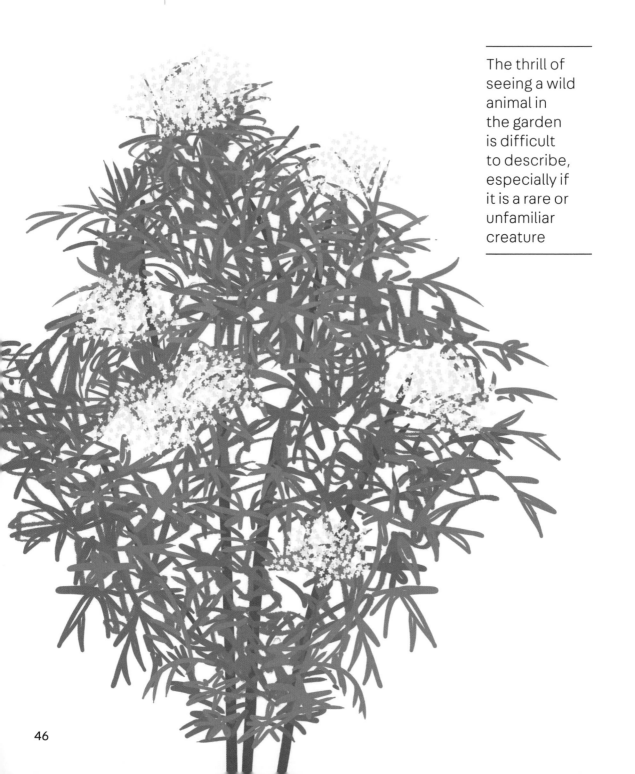

I garden for wildlife. It is the local wildlife's garden, not mine. This is despite my seven years of formal training in horticulture, where the philosophy at the time was based on the idea of humans cultivating and mastering the landscape. Wild animals and plants might fit in, but only if invited or deemed acceptable. I don't follow that doctrine these days, and instead I think of my land as mine only temporarily; I am its custodian for a few years, nothing more. This does not mean it is a nettle patch with only the occasional native tree. Like most domestic plots, my garden is dominated by non-native and cultivated varieties of plant, 'designed in' to demonstrate form and colour, but this process does not exclude the native flora and fauna. In fact, quite the opposite.

Despite the dominance of cultivated ornamental plants, my garden is still a haven for all the local fauna. There are moles in the lawn, roe deer eating the rose flowers, and rabbits climbing the apple trees in winter and stripping the bark – yes, they do climb! On one hand, these are a problem, but on the other, it is a privilege for me to share the space with them. The challenge is to have both, of course, and I can always protect my roses and apples with discreet green wire netting. These native animals and plants are *life*, after all, and a garden should really be about life and promoting natural life cycles. To this end, I stopped using pesticides many years ago.

The thrill of seeing a wild animal in the garden is difficult to describe, especially if it is a rare or unfamiliar creature. And that doesn't apply just to animals either – as anyone will tell you who has had a colony of bee orchids (*Ophrys apifera*) 'arrive' in their lawn. Such moments of wonder are created by the blue-eyed fox cub peering at you through the rhododendrons, or the fledgling green woodpeckers searching for ants on the lawn. I have fond memories of visits to Canadian gardens because of close encounters with bright-red cardinals and striped raccoons, as well as the rarer beavers and fishers. Children in particular find such encounters fascinating, and the positive memories stick. These chance meetings with something wild, unpredictable and uncontrolled are special because they take us away from our routine problems and stresses. They also remind us that we are part of the natural world, not dominant or superior to it. In a strange way, such encounters can be humbling and reassuring, reminding us that our day-to-day problems are not as important as they seem.

So how do we create a biodiversity 'hotspot'? The key is to think like an animal, to work out what it requires. Consider the following:

Water is often vital (see chapters 2 and 7). Do you have space for a small pond or even just a bird bath?

Cover Birds and small mammals, such as the super-cute woodmouse, enjoy thick shrubbery, so surround your plot with shrubs such as elder (*Sambucus*, including the highly attractive black-leaved and pink-flowered varieties such as 'Black Lace'), *Cornus*, *Viburnum*, *Prunus padus* (for European gardens) or *Amelanchier* (for North American gardens).

Vertical greenery Climbers grown on walls and fences will provide nooks and crannies in which insects can hibernate. You don't have to sacrifice colour, so consider *Wisteria*, *Clematis* and climbing (or some of the less vigorous rambling) roses for a wide range of hues.

Open space Animals still need to move through this terrain. They will use your paths, but open grass areas are ideal for viewing foxes, badgers and perhaps even the swoop of a red kite. These can be managed as mini-meadows (see chapter 7) to allow insects to thrive.

Vantage points Consider a small tree, such as *Picea orientalis* 'Skylands', *Pinus leucodermis* 'Satellit' or *Cercidiphyllum japonicum* f. *pendulum*, as a song post for birds such as thrushes and robins. Conifers hold good numbers of small spiders and are favoured as a hunting habitat by secretive species such as goldcrest.

A warm spot A rocky or sandy area will allow reptiles to bask in the early-morning sun in order to warm their blood so that they can become active. You can improve the aesthetics by planting the occasional succulent (such as *Aeonium* 'Zwartkop') or ornamental grass (such as *Pennisetum* 'Fairy Tails' or *Deschampsia cespitosa* 'Golden Dew'). Some specialist insects, such as green tiger beetles, require sandy, stony ground too.

A weedy patch You don't have to let your whole garden become covered in weeds, but you can leave out-of-the-way areas to nature. Adult butterflies will appreciate flowering butterfly bushes

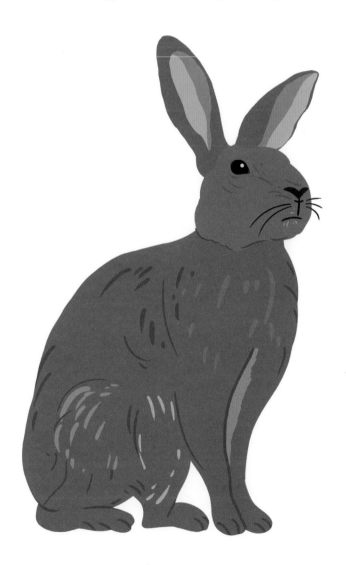

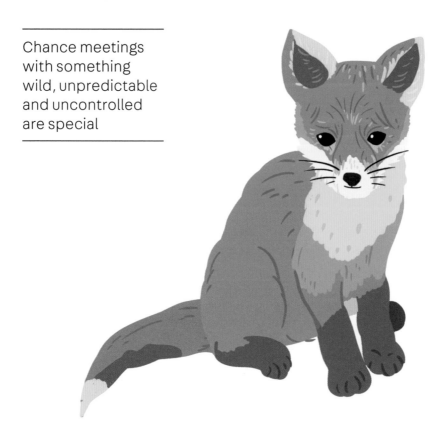

(*Buddleia davidii*) and ice plants (*Hylotelephium spectabile*), for example, but their caterpillars still need nettles (*Urtica dioica*) or grasses (*Agrostis, Dactylis glomerata* and *Elytrigia repens*) to feed on.

Dead wood Although the idea may seem strange, ecologically healthy woodland contains a huge proportion of dead wood. This provides food for the detritivores, those creatures that gain energy by breaking down more complex structures. Dead wood hosts exciting wood-boring beetles, such as the stag beetle, as well as a vast array of fascinating fungi. If you cut back a tree or large shrub, it is a good idea to leave the more substantial branches in a pile somewhere out of the way, for the mini-beasts and fungi to colonize.

Annual flower bonanza A pollinator buzz zone provides a refuelling station for insects. Annual poppies (*Papaver*), cornflowers (*Centaurea cyanus*), love-in-a-mist (*Nigella*), *Cosmos* and many other annuals will provide nectar and pollen for a wide range of insects (see chapter 50).

Bog garden Make the best of a cool, shady spot in your garden by planting *Astilbe* and *Eupatorium cannabinum* to provide a haven for amphibians. Add logs and stones under which animals can hide during very hot or cold periods.

Avoid pesticides and chemicals in general. Despite the fact that some of these are selective (for example, killing only one type of plant), they tend to disrupt the fine ecological balance that can develop in a garden. It's better to tolerate a few pests and let a more complex food chain evolve. This will in itself keep pest numbers in balance.

Connectivity Unless you have a huge garden, your local wildlife will be equally dependent on your neighbours' gardens and on surrounding woods and parkland. It's important that you allow your garden to connect with these. Make holes at the base of fences so that small mammals, such as hedgehogs, can move in and out of 'your' territory.

12 | Digging Deep
Dig or hoe the soil

The American writer and social commentator Meridel Le Sueur once said, 'The body repeats the landscape. They are the source of each other and create each other.' This epitomizes current scientific thinking about the natural world, particularly our relationship with soil and its influence on our health. What the soil and the human body have in common is that there are millions of micro-organisms in both, and these microbial communities may depend on each other to some degree. As our understanding of these communities increases, it is almost as if we are returning to earlier philosophies – the notion of humans being 'made out of clay', or 'the salt of the earth'. Such ideas are a strong metaphor for the link between soil and its life-supporting properties.

Interestingly, both our gut and the soil surrounding plant roots (the rhizosphere) have been described as 'super-organisms' in their own right. We depend on the complex microbial communities in our gut to produce essential amino acids and vitamins, as well as to affect brain function in a more indirect way. Likewise, plants depend on their rhizosphere microbiota for nutrients, hormones and protection against pathogens or environmental stress.

Weed satisfaction

We dig the soil to avoid compaction and to control weeds, especially perennial deep-rooted weeds such as dock (*Rumex*). Once soil has been dug over, weeds can be kept down by frequent hoeing to disrupt the newly germinated smaller weeds. A survey carried out by one of my Ph.D students found that weeding was an activity that divided gardeners right down the middle.[4] Fifty per cent thought it a bore, while the other half considered it the most therapeutic garden activity of all.

What's more, scientists think these 'super-beasts' are related – cousins, as it were. It seems there are direct links between soil 'health' and human gut health. We ingest beneficial microbiota from the soil, but to do so, we must be in regular contact with it, and therein lies the problem. Modern lifestyles limit the opportunity for us to work the soil and expose ourselves to its microbiota. Among indigenous people still living essentially as hunter-gatherers, the gut microbiome is considerably more diverse than it is in those of us who now 'hunt' in the supermarket. This loss of regular direct contact with soil reduces our interaction with beneficial micro-organisms, and the industrialization of agriculture, loss of natural green space and prevalent use of antibiotics, household disinfectants and pesticides all damage natural soil microbiota. This depletion of microbial richness across the board substantially affects human health.

Urban humans, then, must re-establish this link to the soil. We need to get digging, to breathe in the earthy aroma as the soil warms in spring and the microbes get to work. Cultivating the soil and touching it, working it, eating plants that are freshly harvested, all should reinvigorate our stomach-inhabiting microbiota. But as gardeners (or farmers), we must do this carefully, since we want soil that is itself a richly biodiverse, dynamic environment. The soil microbiota is dependent on organic material being returned to the soil and the subsequent activity of invertebrates, such as earthworms, springtails and woodlice. So although I advocate digging (active turning of the soil), don't do it too often. If we think of the soil as a living beast, we must cultivate it carefully. Feed the microbes and create good structure by adding organic compost and mulch. Once you have got on top of the worst weeds, consider a permaculture approach. This means simply hoeing off the weeds every so often, perhaps once a month. By doing so, you will breathe in the beneficial microbiota without disturbing the soil too much.

> Urban humans must re-establish this link to the soil

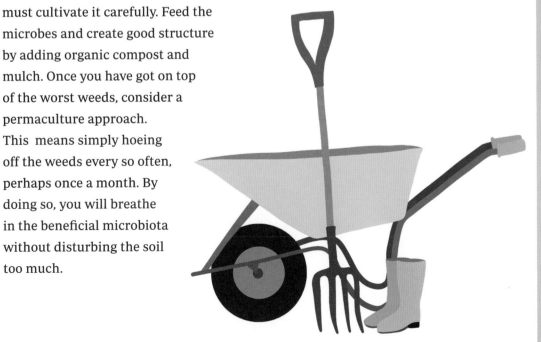

13 | Cool Comfort
Plant a small tree with big leaves

Plants have a strong cooling effect, both by shading hard surfaces (and us) and by absorbing solar energy and using it to convert liquid water in their tissues to vapour. We call this process evapotranspiration.

Planting a tree will keep you and your house cool. It doesn't need to be a fully grown forest giant. For a seating situation in the garden, consider a small tree: redbud (*Cercis canadensis* 'Forest Pansy'), ornamental cherry (*Prunus* Chocolate Ice, also known as 'Matsumae-fuki') or sweetgum (*Liquidambar styraciflua* 'Golden Treasure'), to name but three. There may be other areas that you specifically want to keep cool. In my meadow area, where there is room for a large beast of a tree to reach its full size, I have used the red oak (*Quercus rubra*) to provide shade over a bench. Each leaf of this species is in itself a masterclass in design: about 15–20cm (6–8in) long, evenly serrated and fluttering wonderfully in a light breeze. If you are lucky to get a chilly but bright autumn, it turns a deep red before morphing into a more subtle brown. (For those with a large garden on acid soil, I would instead recommend the scarlet oak, *Q. coccinea*, because it has more reliable red autumn color.)

Those with limited space may wish to plant a medium-sized tree and keep it within bounds through selective pruning now and again. Dramatic large-leaved trees, such as the golden Indian bean tree (*Catalpa bignonioides* 'Aurea') and the foxglove tree (*Paulownia tomentosa*), can be pollarded at head height every two or three years, and will sprout new shoots with umbrella-like leaves that give an instant sun-blocking canopy. The position you choose will depend on when you want sun on the house, and when you do not. A tree just to the west of south (north in the southern hemisphere) will provide

Plants have a strong cooling effect

54

shade from mid-afternoon onwards, so you could get shade on the house just as air temperatures start to peak, while still enjoying strong light during the morning and over lunch.

Don't forget climbers and wall shrubs. One of my Ph.D students found that plants such as honeysuckle (*Lonicera periclymenum*), jasmine (*Jasminum officinale*) and *Fuchsia* were particularly effective at cooling brick walls (see below). All have lovely flowers in yellow/cream, white and red respectively, and the first two have the bonus of delicious evening scent. If space is limited, consider annual climbers; nasturtium (*Tropaeolum*), sweet pea (*Lathyrus*) and morning glory (*Convolvulus*) are all rampant and can cover a wall quickly before the first frost conveniently 'disposes' of them for you.

Thermal comfort and the wallet

Plants keep buildings cool in summer, but they also insulate against heat loss in winter. In controlled studies, my Ph.D student Jane Taylor showed that plants grown against a brick wall reduced energy loss in winter by about one third.[5] Plants are natural insulators, and can save us money by reducing our reliance on mechanical air conditioning in summer and on central heating in winter. Both aspects will help in our fight against the climate crisis by lowering carbon dioxide emissions.

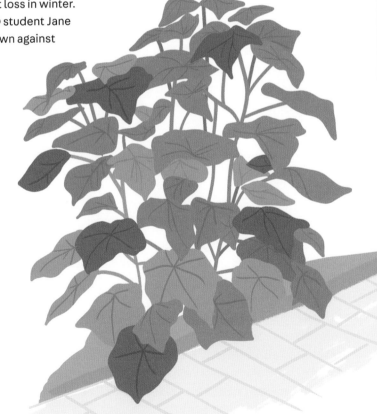

14 Inky and Spooky
Grow purple carrots, full of anthocyanins

Carrots are orange, right? Well, most are, but not all. The wild carrot (*Daucus carota*) has a thin, pale cream-coloured root that tastes somewhat bitter. The cultivated orange carrot (*D.c.* subsp. *sativus*) is a product of many years of selection and breeding, carried out most enthusiastically by the Dutch, resulting in a larger, sweeter, more consistently shaped root crop. But you do also get white, yellow, red, black and – yes – purple varieties. Carrots are thought to have originated in central Asia and were first cultivated in Afghanistan, where the purple carrot was eaten and also used in the dyeing of royal gowns.

Modern purple carrot varieties include 'Purple Haze', 'Purple Sun', 'Dragon Purple' and 'Deep Purple'. Children love strong colours, and talking to them about unusual carrots can get them interested in growing and (fingers crossed) eating them, too. Some seed

Which are the healthiest carrots?

All carrots are healthy, but by eating a mixture of colours you could be widening the range of beneficial compounds (nutraceuticals) you are ingesting. The colour of a carrot depends on the proportion of pigments in its tissues. These pigments and other compounds affect its dietary contributions, so different cultivars provide different health benefits. Purple carrots are full of anthocyanins, purple pigments with antioxidant properties that protect our cells from damage. Thus purple carrots are linked to protection against various forms of cancer and heart disease (they particularly help to protect artery cells from injury, thus potentially stopping hardening of the arteries). They may have 30 times the anthocyanins of standard orange carrots. But the benefits don't stop there. Purple carrots are rich in other chemical compounds, known as phenolics, and in falcarinol, which also helps heart health and inhibits the formation of cancer cells. By contrast, yellow and orange carrots contain more carotene and xanthophyll pigments, and these are linked to maintaining eye health (see page 59), including a reduced incidence of cataracts.

The litmus test

Interestingly, the prevalent molecular form of some anthocyanins can depend on pH. They are red in acidic conditions and blue-purple in alkaline solutions, so – theoretically, at least – we could use purple carrots as living litmus paper. In fact, the original litmus paper used dyes extracted from lichens (a living structure that is a combination of a fungus and an alga), so using plants to test pH is not as fanciful as it might seem.

Purple carrots are linked to protection against various forms of cancer and heart disease merchants produce packets of carrot seed that include white, orange, red, yellow and purple varieties, and it is great fun to sow these with children and wait to see what colours you pull from the earth a couple of months later. Unearth two consecutive carrots of the same colour and shout 'Bingo!'

The country or region of origin of a plant can give clues about its cultivation. Exploring and understanding a plant's background (its environmental eco-physiology) can be fun, and it helps us to place and manage it in the garden or house. The clue with carrot is its origin in arid Afghanistan. That means these plants like free-draining, sandy soil, and abhor heavy, sticky clay. So if your ground is mainly clay, grow your carrots in a large container of loose, free-draining (peat-free) growing medium.

Sow carrots over a number of weeks to spread out harvesting – otherwise it will be boiled carrots, baked carrots, stir-fried carrots, carrot salad, carrot cake, carrot flan, carrot crumble and carrot surprise all in a single week. Root vegetables do store well, but it's still a good idea to avoid a 'glut and famine' scenario as best you can. Carrots are normally sown outdoors in spring or summer and harvested throughout summer and autumn. If you have space in the garden, early varieties can be sown outdoors as early as late winter and protected under a plastic or glass cloche. You may need to thin the plants out (remove some seedlings to increase the distance between them), as they will compete for space, water and nutrients. Be sure to discard any waste seedlings well away from the crop; the number one pest of carrots is carrot root fly, and they home in on the smell of injured carrot from far and wide.

Carrots and night vision

'Eat your carrots and you will be able to see in the dark' is one of those phrases often used by parents trying to encourage their children to eat healthily. But is it true? Actually, carrots do have a role in maintaining good eye health. Vitamin A, which they contain in abundance, keeps the cornea clear and is involved in the formation of rhodopsin, a protein in the eye that is linked with vision in low light. But it's an exaggeration to say that eating lots of carrots will suddenly make the nocturnal world visible.

It's not apparent exactly where that much-used claim originates. It may relate to the fact that 'night-fighter' pilots during World War II were encouraged to improve their night vision by eating more healthily and looking after their bodies. At a time when 'luxury' overseas foods were scarce, eating homegrown staple crops, such as carrots and potatoes, was a necessity for a healthy, balanced diet. Consequently, promoting the virtues of such food was part of the war propaganda.

Indeed, the promotion of carrots may have been closely linked to a specific piece of propaganda. The Allies' development of a new form of radar embedded directly into the body of a fighter aircraft (rather than placed on, and functioning from, the ground) allowed the night fighters to close in on enemy bombers more effectively. It is said that the Allies tried to explain through propaganda the resulting rapid increase in enemy bombers being shot down at night by putting it down to the increased consumption of carrots by their pilots, rather than any new technology. Whether the opposing forces believed that is anyone's guess.

15 | Success with Succulents
Keep indoor succulents

Perhaps because of their low maintenance requirements, succulents tend to bring out the plant physiologist in me, rather than my inner gardener. They might be easy to manage, but that is only because of their amazing capacity to withstand all the extremes of temperature and drought that nature can throw at them. The more you understand how these extraordinary plants work, the more intriguing they become.

The ingenuity of succulents parallels that of the villain in a spy movie

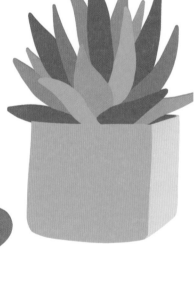
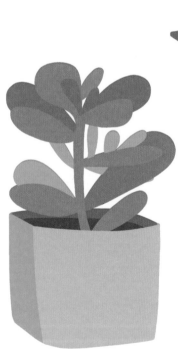
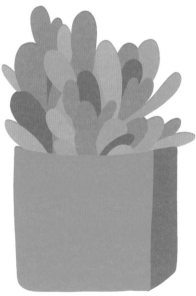

Succulents store water in their leaves and stem, and that 'plastic' appearance is the shrink-wrap they use to retain this hard-won moisture. They possess thick, waxy skins (cuticles) that stop water evaporating from the surface, and have developed unusual colours to protect the leaves from overheating and from the strong ultraviolet light of the desert. *Aeonium* 'Zwartkop', for example, is almost black, and *Cotyledon orbiculata* silvery blue. The 'power source' of these botanical curiosities – their chloroplasts, which harvest photons from the sun and split the water molecule that gives them the energy to 'build' their food – are buried deep in the tissues of the leaf or stem. Their ingenuity parallels that of the villain in a spy movie. Biological power plants, energy transformers and 'secret-formula' chemical labs are hidden in a labyrinth of pipes and vascular passageways. The high-tech biochemicals they produce are all about hanging on to precious water molecules despite the searing heat, and deterring enemy pathogens from attacking their inner workings.

Aloe vera, with its wide range of cosmetic and antimicrobial applications (its gel-like sap and latex are both used), is one of the most famous succulents. But there are some succulents that you don't even know are there. These are the living stones of South Africa: species of *Lithops*. Being the spitting image of a typical seaside pebble, these plants protect themselves from hungry mouths by blending into the desert gravel, and conserve moisture through their convex, space-age 'biome' shape. Place them on a sunny windowsill and they will eventually expand into a colony of 'pebbles'.

The symmetry of some succulents is a wonder. *Crassula* 'Buddha's Temple' looks like some ancient Aztec artefact, with its mesmerizing pyramidal tiers. Then there are the things that look as if they have wandered off a coral reef. This includes the aptly named *Aloe vera* 'Starfish', *Ceropegia woodii* 'Silver Glory', the crown cactus (*Rebutia arenacea*) and the towering *Euphorbia trigona*. All are fantastic shapes and great talking points.

Health Benefit
Positive Affect

Nature can provide small moments of joy (positive affect), but its capacity to do this frequently helps to improve our overall mood. Strong positive mood is an antidote to certain mental-health problems, so essentially gardening can give you joy that in itself helps to build in resilience to mental-health problems. Positive affect is being increasingly studied in the field of psychology, as is the way its individual elements – among them happiness, good mood, optimism, humour, enthusiasm and love – influence long-term mental health.

Positive affect can be difficult to quantify scientifically owing to the diverse components that culminate in a positive state of mind, but in terms of engagement with nature, I see it manifest itself as the momentary excitement we feel when we notice something stunning or unusual. I describe it as the 'wow factor' – those moments that elicit emotions such as amazement, admiration, awe and surprise.

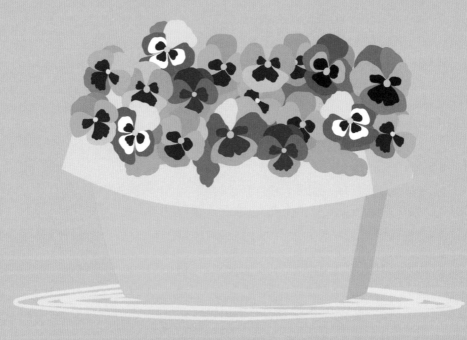

At a larger landscape scale, this is the wonder we might experience when we reach the brow of a hill and see a beautiful valley laid out below. It is not necessarily passive; this is the emotion we seek when we watch a storm rolling in over the ocean and the breakers pounding the harbour wall. Studies have also linked more positive experiences to locations with more diverse wildlife.[6]

Positive affect is democratic, and there should be no hierarchy. For some, the effect is elicited by seeing the rare golden oriole (a very flashy yellow-and-black bird, made all the more magical by its rarity in northern Europe), but for others it is the 'common' robin bobbing about by the doorstep. The joy such encounters give is very personal.

Positive affect in a garden context can also come in many guises: the myriad lustrous hues of a single *Dahlia* petal; the taste of a freshly plucked raspberry, peach or mango; the amazing harmony of the famous White Garden at Sissinghurst in Kent or the vibrant displays of azaleas at Biltmore in North Carolina. We can access positive, uplifting emotions even in winter by seeing enormous, dagger-like icicles hanging off the tips of an old weeping willow (*Salix*), for example, or low sunlight illuminating the blood-red bark of a Tibetan cherry (*Prunus serrula*).

Psychologists are still exploring the many ways positive affect can manifest itself in the landscape, and indeed it may be about not just momentary pleasure, but also longer-term relationships with landscapes and nature. Such research is in its infancy, but it could relate to concepts that have been around for a long time in horticulture and landscape architecture – not least what is meant by *genius loci* or 'sense of place'. This term has been used for centuries to signify a special ambience, resonance or positive emotion provided by a particular landscape.

16 | Colour on the Move
Plant *Buddleia* for butterflies

The butterfly bush (*Buddleia davidii*) is the fast-food outlet of the insect world. It will attract butterflies and other pollinating insects from miles around. It was the first plant I ever bought for my parents' garden, precisely so that I could bring in more butterflies (at the age of nine I wanted to be an entomologist, not a horticulturalist, but this plant set me on the latter path). The plant is strikingly attractive, with its long panicles of pale mauve, purple-blue, white and sometimes pink flowers. Golden or variegated cultivars are now becoming common, and extend the season of interest through their attractive foliage. *Buddleia* can, however, be dismissed because of its invasiveness. It will quite happily take over old railway sidings and disused gravel quarries, where it is well suited to the warm microclimate and free-draining soil.

Not all plants are aptly named, but the butterfly bush certainly is. A single specimen can host 30–40 feeding butterflies at any one time. *Buddleia* is particularly attractive to butterflies (or, at least, the larger species, whose long probosces can reach the nectaries at the back of the flower) because of the quality of its nectar. *Buddleia* nectar contains the sugars fructose and glucose, but is especially high in sucrose, and it is this 'high-octane' fuel that draws in the butterflies. The volume of nectar available in each flower is limited, though, and the butterfly must move around the bush to maximize its sugar dose. That is why they tend to stay on one plant for some time.

> *Buddleia* nectar is especially high in sucrose, and it is this 'high-octane' fuel that draws in the butterflies

Butterflies are the epitome of grace and beauty, and indeed the antithesis of anything creepy-crawly. Their languid wingbeats and lack of apparent urgency as they flit from one flower to the next are relaxing for us to view. But in

What's in a name?

Our familiarity with and feelings for butterflies are mirrored in the common names we give them. Awe and wonder at their majestic brilliance are expressed in the names of the purple emperor, blue-spotted emperor, red admiral and Camberwell beauty, and links to other animals that we admire can be seen in the swallowtail, peacock, blue albatross, small tortoiseshell and zebra longwing. Other names show how their colours (brimstone, blue morpho, turquoise jewel) or markings (comma, paper kite) reflect everyday objects.

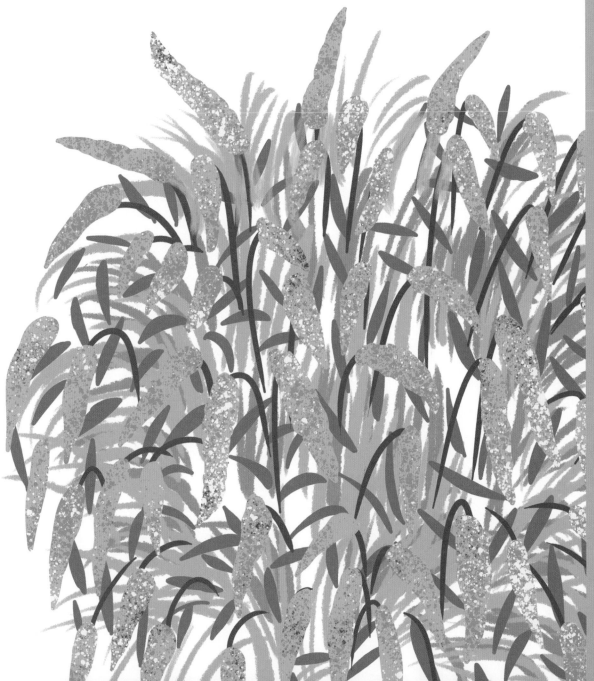

HEALTH BENEFIT: **BIOPHILIA**

65

Other plants to attract butterflies

As well as *Buddleia*, a number of plants are rich in nectar and have the appropriate flower forms to bring in the butterflies. These include the flat 'pin-cushion' florets of the ice plant (*Hylotelephium spectabile*), the original species of which has better nectar supplies than some of the more recent cultivars. The light, ethereal *Verbena bonariensis* has tall stems topped with deep mauve flowers. In warmer climates, species of *Lantana* are the butterfly plant of choice, with bicoloured flowers – orange with pink or red with yellow – that are also attractive in themselves. As with *Buddleia*, be careful where you use them; they are considered invasive weeds in some places, including Hawaii.

We must also consider food plants for the caterpillars. Wherever you can, leave space for 'wild' plants, such as ivy (*Hedera*), holly (*Ilex*), lady's smock (*Cardamine pratense*), nettle (*Urtica dioica*) and a range of meadow grasses, to allow these beautiful insects to complete their life cycle.

Watching butterflies is a distracting activity that allows us to switch off temporarily from our daily pressures and stresses

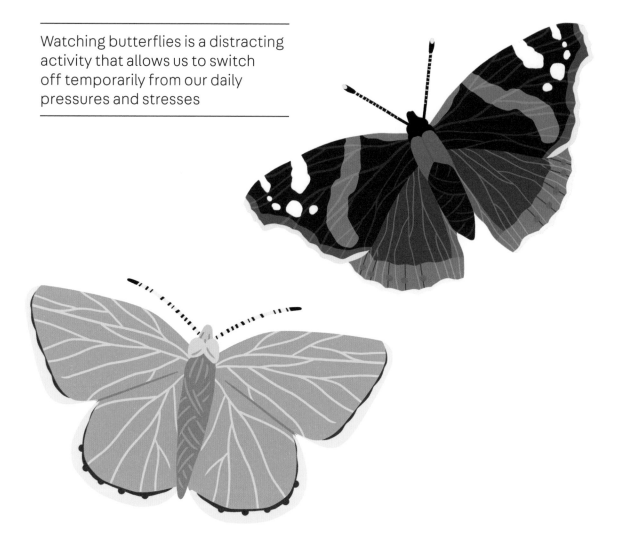

reality they are surprisingly strong fliers – hence the requirement for those sugar-laden drinks – and some, such as the monarch and the painted lady, undertake lengthy migrations. Butterflies are equally famous for the colour of their wings, and most species are bright and bold in their coloration. Some possess 'eye spots' in their patterning, and when they open their wings the sudden appearance of these eyes scares off predators such as birds or small mammals.

Watching butterflies is a distracting activity that allows us to switch off temporarily from our daily pressures and stresses. These carefree moments are important to relax the body, find respite from mental fatigue and reset our priorities. Such iconic insects typify the natural world and our love of it. Their apparent fragility and short lifespan should make us realize how precious life is, and remind us to make the most of it. They are increasingly representative of a fragile ecosystem, too, and of the fact that we – as now effectively custodians of the natural world – must manage it better and conserve its complexity. In many ways, butterflies are the archetypical biophilic species; we love them, find their colours infinitely fascinating and are entranced by their flight across our path when we are out in the garden or on a country walk.

A trick of the light

Some butterflies have reflective wing scales, cells that reflect and refract light rather than possessing their own pigments. These shine and dazzle as the angle of sunlight changes, and what appears dark russet-brown can morph into sapphire or amethyst with the flick of a wing.

Perfume from the Veld

Introduce pelargoniums for their scent

I can't look at a red-flowered *Pelargonium*, especially if it is growing in a terracotta pot, and not be reminded of charming villages by the Mediterranean. To me, red pelargoniums go hand in hand with steep, cobbled alleyways, sunshine and the balconies of whitewashed Spanish villas. But the true home of the *Pelargonium* is actually South Africa (although see page 71). Both Spain and South Africa have Mediterranean climates, meteorologically speaking – mild, wet winters and hot, dry summers – so it is easy to see why these plants do well around the shores of the Mediterranean. As with many other plants from Mediterranean climate zones, pelargoniums are endowed with aromatic essential oils (phytoncides) that discourage attack by herbivores (both mammals and insects), but also provide our cells with a degree of protection from damaging biochemical reactions (see pages 172–3).

Pelargonium is a very popular bedding plant, one that is frequently planted out in massed ranks in early summer, in well-prepared flower beds. But you would not necessarily know this, because in garden centres these plants – commonly sold in trays of six or eight – are marketed as 'geraniums'. If you venture to the herbaceous perennial section of the garden centre, you will find other geraniums, but they look quite different from the first lot. These herbaceous perennial geraniums, with their symmetrical, button-like flowers, are the true botanical *Geranium* (sometimes called hardy geraniums or cranesbills). The *Pelargonium*, on the other hand, is not really a geranium at all, but the two types were once classified together, so the name 'geranium' has stuck, despite being reclassified as long ago as 1789.

Most people are familiar with the bedding *Pelargonium* types, which are treated as half-hardy annuals (grown under glasshouse

Leaf power

Some of the species and scented-leaf varieties of Pelargonium may not have the showy, 'in your face' flowers of the other groups, but the intricate shapes and hues of their petals make them every bit as interesting. Many are tough little native species of southern and eastern Africa, and they have varied and attractive foliage – not least because of the pleasant scents their essential oils (phytoncides) give off. Lemon is a prevalent scent, as the cultivar 'Citronella' testifies; the many other aromas include peppermint, apple and woody balsam. It is precisely these aromatic chemicals that scientists believe provide the beneficial effects for the human body.

protection and planted out in spring after the last frost). These include the zonal pelargonium, so called because of the 'zone' of darker green or purple that runs through each leaf. The zonals have flowers in a range of pink, white, red, salmon and orange hues. Being bedding plants, they adapt well to containers, and flower consistently and strongly throughout the summer. Other pelargonium types also make great container plants. The ivy-leaved group (derived from *P. peltatum*) can be used to trail out of hanging baskets or over the lip of a tub. Notable characters in this group include 'Harvard', with vibrant, true-red flowers; 'Amethyst', a curious purple-pink; and 'Joan of Arc', which has pure white flowers with two or three red inkspots on the upper petals.

I see most other types of *Pelargonium* as transitional plants, by which I mean they can be kept indoors in a well-lit location over winter, then moved after the last frost to the patio or close to other outdoor seating. Essentially, when we are outside, they are outside. In summer they will enjoy any suntrap you can provide for them. Indeed, most *Pelargonium* species are best handled as perennial, 'conservatory-type' plants, kept in their own pots throughout; with a bit of luck they will provide joy for many, many years – as long as you remember to move them in line with the seasons. It is these perennial, conservatory selections that I truly associate with South Africa, although they come from a surprising range of habitats, ranging from the Western Cape coast to the mountains. Within this

Pelargoniums are endowed
with aromatic essential
oils that provide our cells
with a degree of protection
from damaging biochemical
reactions

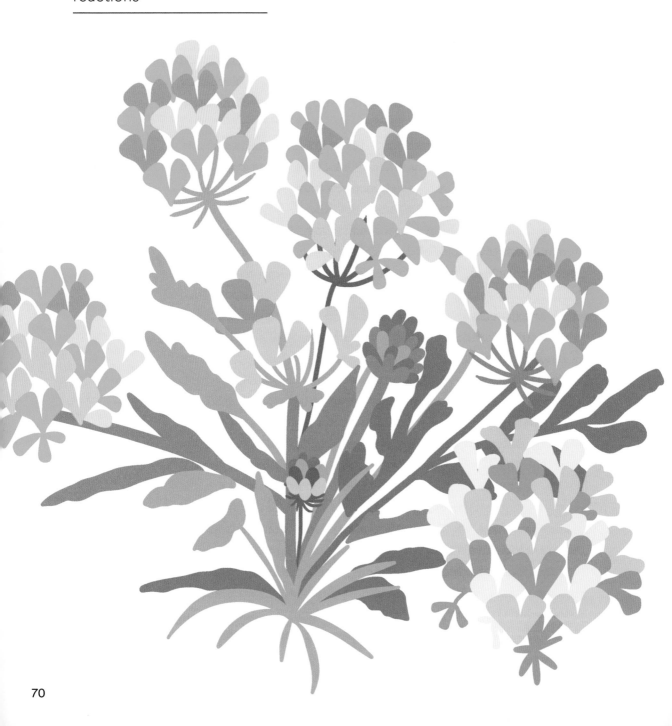

category are the pansy-faced 'Angel' group, the so-called decoratives (aren't most *Pelargonium* decorative?), the regals and the scented-leaf types.

The regals are a useful group to start with if you have not grown *Pelargonium* before. Basically, all they need is frost-free conditions. They start to flower quite early in spring and, if given potassium-based liquid fertilizer as they grow, will continue to flower well throughout the summer. They have some of the most colourful flowers of all the pelargoniums, with pure white at one end of the spectrum and almost black at the other. Often the petals have two tones, or they may be of one colour with a fringe in a contrasting hue. My personal favourites include 'Fareham', two-tone purple; 'Lord Bute', maroon-purple with red lining the edge; and 'Joan Morf', morphing between various shades of pink and white.

Branching out

Pelargonium are associated with South Africa, but small numbers of species come from East Africa, Madagascar, Turkey, Socotra, Yemen and Iraq. Species are also found on the islands of Tristan da Cunha and St Helena, thousands of miles off the west coast of Africa. More surprisingly, a small number of species are found in Australia and New Zealand. Two theories have been put forward to explain how these essentially African plants reached such far-flung locations:

1 The ancestors of today's species lived on the Earth's single supercontinent, Gondwana, and when this split up, plants evolved differently on the separate continents as they moved apart, forming new species.

2 Plants can disperse over great distances thanks to their seed. For example, seeds carried on driftwood or in birds' feathers can help plants colonize new areas.

Since *Pelargonium* is a relatively young plant family in evolutionary terms, botanists think the second theory is the more likely explanation in this case.

18 | Chill Out with Cool Colours
Choose blue, white and green plants

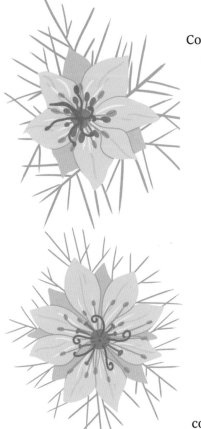

Cool colours (greens, blues and whites) are deemed calming, while hot colours (reds, oranges and yellows) are seen as exhilarating. Research studies tend to bear this out when it comes to flower and foliage colour. Cool colours are relaxing and create harmony in a planting composition. Sometimes less is more, and limiting yourself to two or three colours can provide better synergy and bring out the subtle effects of individual plants more effectively.

If you have a semi-shady corner in the garden, or want to cover an unsightly wall or shed, consider planting a mix of small trees, shrubs, herbaceous plants and annuals to create a harmonious effect with cool colours. If you have a lightly shaded spot, choose one of the green Japanese maples (*Acer palmatum*). The types with dissected leaves, such as 'Emerald Lace', have a refined, dainty appeal. To provide a little contrast through a bolder, stronger leaf shape you might add *Hydrangea paniculata* 'Limelight', with its large plumes of pale lime-green flowers maturing over time to white and sometimes pink. In a similar vein is *Viburnum opulus* 'Roseum', with its balls of sterile flowers in pale green or cream. Consider planting one of the mock oranges (such as *Philadelphus* 'Beauclerk') to add to the white floral theme, but also bring the luscious scent of orange to the mix. For a delicate late summer effect, *Fuchsia* 'Hawkshead' has simple white bell-like flowers. Ivy can be used to screen a wall, and here *Hedera hibernica* 'Hamilton' stands out with its distinctive leaf shape, providing an attractive mid-green facade.

Herbaceous plants can be dispersed among the shrubs, or positioned slightly in front to take centre stage when they flower. Continuing the white theme, you can achieve early flowers with the Christmas rose (*Helleborus niger*) in late winter and the pheasant's-eye daffodil (*Narcissus poeticus*) in spring. *Dicentra spectabilis* 'Alba' provides an arch of heart-shaped flowers in early summer, and this can be followed by *Phlox paniculata* 'White Admiral' and *Physostegia virginiana* 'Alba'. ('Alba' means white, so you will come across this word a lot when searching for white flowers.) Maintain late summer interest with *Anemone × hybrida* 'Honorine Jobert', its anthers creating an amber wheel at the heart of each flower, which is reminiscent of the pheasant's-eye daffodil. Bold-textured *Hosta* provide ground cover throughout the growing season and add to the relaxing mantle of green.

White and green alone are both dramatic and soothing, but blue can be added for a different effect. *Veronica spicata* 'Royal Candles', with its deep-blue spires, will do well in a more open position near

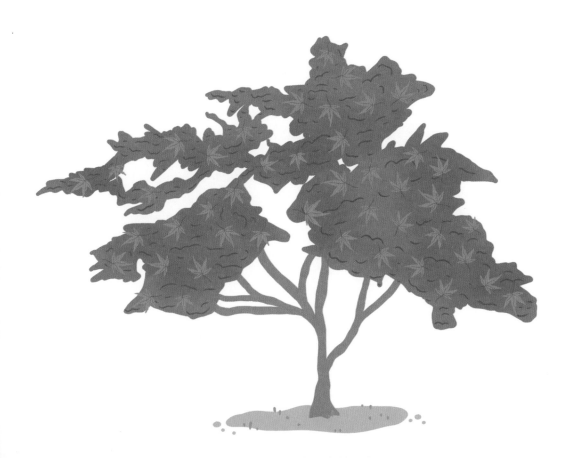

the front of the border. Jacob's ladder (*Polemonium caeruleum*) has a mauve-blue flower and fern-like foliage, while *Tradescantia virginiana* 'Blue 'n' Gold' throws up strap-like green-gold leaves set off with blue button flowers. Finally for the perennials, I would squeeze in *Aquilegia coerulea* (or *caerulea*), from the Rocky Mountains, for its blue-and-white flowers.

If there is any space left, add some annuals and biennials. In fact, even if there isn't any space, placing a few pots in front of the border gives you an excuse to grow more plants and provides additional summer interest. The star-white flowers of the white Beacon *Impatiens* (busy Lizzie) will simply glow out from a background of deep-green foliage. White snapdragons, such as *Antirrhinum* 'Sonnet White', have a fresh appeal, and *Nicotiana* Cuba strain comes in pure-white or lime-green flowers, so either will fit into the scheme. The flowers on the foxglove *Digitalis* 'Pam's Split' are not pure white, having a deep-purple centre, but this is not intrusive enough for us to exclude it from the mix.

For the blues we have the classic *Lobelia*; *L. erinus* 'Crystal Palace' is deep blue, and although *L.e.* 'Cambridge Blue' is not Cambridge blue at all, it is a very attractive denim-blue, and warrants its place on that basis. A plant that prefers a bit more sun is *Nigella damascena* 'Moody Blues', but I would take the chance and include it here. If you want the best of both worlds, the amusingly named *Viola hybrida* 'Sorbet Yesterday Today & Tomorrow' has flowers that come out white but after two or three days turn mid-blue. It's fairly uncommon – and thus spectacular – to see a variety of hues all on the same plant.

Green pain relief

We can thank the willow tree (*Salix*) for the invention of the painkilling drug aspirin (active ingredient: acetylsalicylic acid), but it is worth mentioning that pain can also be reduced simply by observing the willow tree. The healthcare design researcher Roger Ulrich was working with medical colleagues in the United States with the aim of improving the comfort of patients after gallbladder surgery. He observed that patients who were placed in rooms with views of nearby parkland recovered more quickly than those in otherwise similar rooms with no green views. Those patients also needed fewer analgesics (painkilling drugs) and tended to have more positive comments on their medical notes. The medical authorities were happy too, since these findings meant they could reduce their drug bills.

White and green alone are both dramatic and soothing

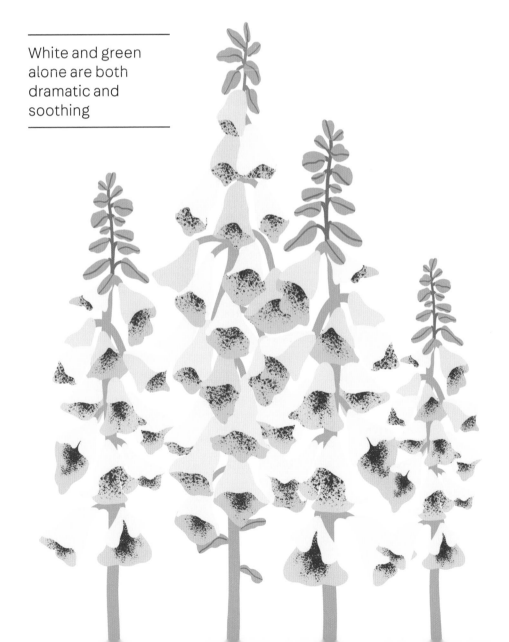

Health Benefit
Healthy Eating

Even before humans were humans, we had an intimate relationship with plants, because we needed to eat them. Most primates and apes rely on plants, with only occasional forays into insects for some, to provide a protein boost. Of our near cousins, it is only the chimpanzees and bonobos that actively hunt and eat other mammals. So, despite our craving for queueing at burger stands in shopping malls, it is really plants that are essential for our nutrition. Plants provide us with carbohydrates, proteins, certain fats, fibre, essential minerals and vitamins. Some plants, though, furnish us with these substances in greater quantities, or in forms that may be particularly beneficial to maintain healthy cells or organ function. These so-called superfood plants are linked to enhanced 'antioxidant' behaviour, where certain compounds inhibit the activity of free radical ions (oxidants) at a cellular level.[7] Not only does this help to keep our cells intact, but also in terms of our whole physiology it promotes immunity from disease.

A regular, balanced diet (that is to say, one that contains a wide variety of beneficial compounds) is encouraged in order for us to improve immunity and resist the chronic diseases that are associated with long-term wear and tear of the body (heart disease, cancer, diabetes, stroke, bowel inflammation and so on). A short list of plants with associated benefits is given opposite. By growing your own food, you guarantee that it is fresh. This not only gives a more delightful flavour, but also means that the beneficial compounds have not degraded before you eat them.

Plant type	High in	Health benefit
Brassicas (cabbages)	Folate, fibre, vitamin C, zinc, calcium, iron, magnesium, carotenoids	Help to prevent heart disease, type 2 diabetes and cancer
Red and black berries	Vitamins, minerals, fibre, antioxidants	Help to prevent heart disease, cancer and other inflammatory conditions
Legumes (peas and pulses)	Vitamin B, minerals, protein, fibre	Regulate type 2 diabetes management, blood pressure, cholesterol and weight (because they make you feel full)
Nuts and seeds	Fibre, vegetarian protein and heart-healthy fats, anti-inflammatories, antioxidants	Help to prevent heart disease
Garlic	Manganese, vitamin C, vitamin B6, selenium, sulphur, fibre	Regulates cholesterol, blood pressure and immune response Helps to prevent cancer
Olive	Monounsaturated fatty acids and polyphenolic compounds, antioxidants such as vitamins E and K	Reduces inflammation and cellular damage from oxidative stress Helps to prevent heart disease and diabetes
Ginger	Antioxidants, such as gingerol	Regulates nausea and reduces pain from acute and chronic inflammatory conditions Helps to prevent heart disease, dementia and certain cancers
Avocado	Nutrients, fibre, vitamins, minerals and healthy fats Oleic acid is the predominant monounsaturated fat	Helps to prevent inflammation, heart disease, diabetes, metabolic syndromes and certain types of cancer
Sweet potato	Nutrients, including potassium, fibre, vitamins A and C, carotenoids	Improves blood sugar control in those with type 2 diabetes

19 | Grow your Own Superfoods
Cultivate the common cabbage

We have already touched on a number of superfoods (see chapters 9 and 14, and pages 76–7), but there is one vegetable that really takes the crown, and that is the leafy common cabbage and its relatives, including cauliflower, Brussels sprouts, kohlrabi, kale and broccoli. Botanically speaking, all these plants are *Brassica oleracea*.

Some cabbages are an acquired taste, but stick with them, especially when encouraging children to eat them (little and often works better than large 'doses' at a time). Older children and young teenagers often shun cabbages, but may return to them later, once the palate matures. Cabbages are connected with a wide range of health benefits, of which a few are listed opposite.

Cabbages can be harvested almost all year round, but if space is limited, you can select varieties that are particularly suited to your needs, whether that be for cool summer salads or tasty winter soups. If you have a spare piece of soil or, even better, a raised bed full of fertile compost, it's easy to cultivate a small crop of cabbages. Alternatively, consider growing them individually in large tubs. The ball of leaves that is eventually harvested is called the 'head' or 'crown', and can be 40cm (16in) in diameter, so a decent space is required to allow it to develop fully.

Cabbages are known as 'gross feeders', which means they require a growing medium that is very fertile. These and other leafy vegetables require good quantities of the plant nutrient nitrogen, and this tends to be high in organic composts. The key with nitrogen is to feed the plant during the growing phase, a little and often. So, in addition to growing the plants in a nutritious compost, you can fertilize them as they grow with a liquid feed.

Health benefit	How it works
Cancer prevention	Through regulating cell behaviour, encouraging 'correct' cell division and avoiding 'incorrect' growth of tumour cells. Commonly occurring compounds such as sulforaphane, lupeol and sinigrin stimulate enzyme activity that inhibits the growth of tumour cells. Human cultures that eat cabbage regularly are linked with the lowest rates of colon cancer.
Anti-inflammatory processes	Glutamine and anthocyanins (the latter especially in red cabbage) are anti-inflammatory compounds and help to reduce joint pain as well as fever, allergies and inflammation of the skin.
Boosting immunity	Antioxidants such as vitamin C (which reduce the activity of free radicals), and enzymes and prebiotics that help with gut function, strengthen the immune system.
Skin and hair conditioning	Through the action of sulphur and silica, both of which are common in the plant.
Conditioning of the nervous system	Vitamins B and K, which are found in high levels in red cabbage, help the nervous system. Vitamin K fortifies the myelin sheaths that surround the nerve endings, and vitamin B restores nerve cells and regulates blood supply. Such protective properties help to offset Alzheimer's disease and other forms of dementia later in life.
Lowering cholesterol	Phytosterols block the adherence of 'damaging' cholesterol from high-fat foods in the digestive tract. Cholesterol is also present in bile acid, and the fibre in cabbages helps to excrete the excess.
Providing omega-3 fatty acids	Additional regulation against inflammatory diseases, including cardiovascular disease and arthritis.
Improving bone strength	Minerals, especially calcium and magnesium, aid bone construction and help us to avoid osteoporosis in later life.
Supporting colon health	Protects and cleans the colon by sustaining key gut bacteria and encouraging the passage of food.
Repairing stomach ulcers	S-methylmethionine eases the pain of a stomach ulcer and L-glutamine improves blood flow to injured areas.

You can buy concentrated liquid fertilizers from the garden centre, but you might try making your own. Leave 1kg (1¼lb) fresh nettle leaves (*Urtica dioica*) in a bucket of water (10 litres/about 2½ gallons) for two weeks and you will end up with a concentrate that is high in nitrogen. (Use thick gloves when dealing with the nettles – they have a nasty sting.) Dilute this liquid 1:10 with water and feed the cabbages once a week as their heads begin to develop and expand. Some specialist growers, who compete at flower shows to produce the biggest cabbage for that year, swear that adding beer as liquid fertilizer further enhances growth, but others argue that the best outcome is to have a smaller cabbage and drink the beer yourself.

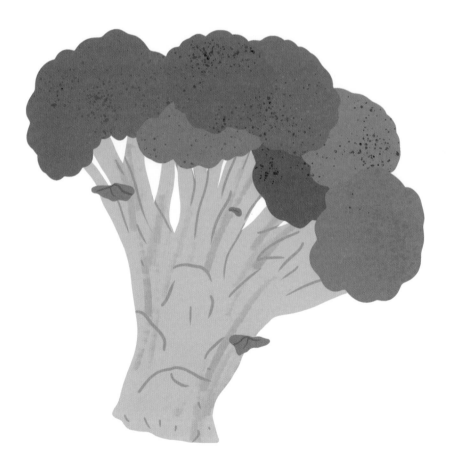

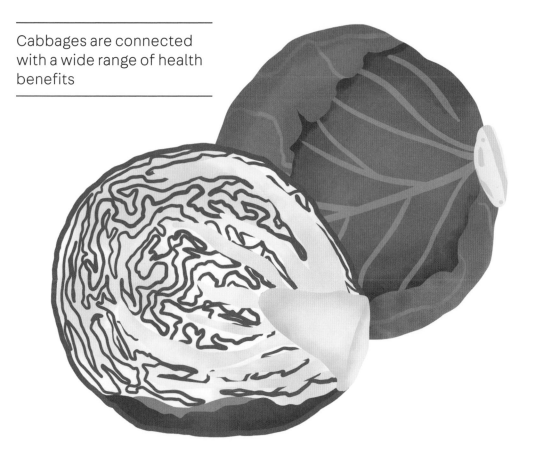

Cabbages are connected with a wide range of health benefits

For the more adventurous

The leafy 'ball' cabbages are the types to start with. Varieties such as 'Hispi' (which is harvested in spring or summer), 'Tundra' (a Savoy-type cabbage harvested in winter) and the compact, pointed 'Pixie' (spring harvest) are ideal. Don't forget to try your luck with the red-leaved ones, too, such as 'Red Jewel'.

Once you gain confidence, consider brassicas that form an edible floret head (cauliflower) or offshoots (Brussels sprouts). For cauliflowers, try 'Galleon' (spring harvest), 'Nessie' (summer harvest) and, to continue the aquatic theme, 'Moby Dick' for early winter. If you fancy something more colourful, 'Graffiti' has purple florets (which

are generally called curds in a cauliflower).

The sprouts in Brussels sprouts are mini cabbage heads. They form in the axils of the main stem (the angle between the top of the leaf stalk and the stem), and those that form early, near the base of the plant, are the first to be harvested. This should be done when they are about 2cm (nearly 1in) in diameter and the leaves are still tightly furled. Sprouts are harvested in the autumn and winter, and some varieties require exposure to frost to bring out the best flavour; others can be harvested in late summer. Cultivars to look out for are 'Maximus' and 'Clodius'.

20 | Plant by Numbers
Use plants that have regular shapes and symmetry

For us to gain the greatest health benefits from nature, nature must 'make sense' to us. This is a component of the Attention Restoration theory (see pages 9 and 122–3). For humans to benefit from the relaxing effect of nature, and for it to restore the brain's capacity to do work (direct attention), the experiences of nature must align (be compatible) with our understanding of the natural world. This is one reason why it's important to introduce children to the natural world at an early age, and encourage them to learn about its positive and negative elements during their development. We view nature differently depending on our early experiences and on the social environment and culture in which we are brought up. Attitudes to natural features and phenomena can be polarized – for example, our feelings about birds such as seagulls.

Our 'nurture' (learned) influences can manifest themselves as preferences for different types of garden or design style. Some people love informality, whereas others desire symmetry and neatness. Some want the familiar and may adopt a style similar to the one their parents enjoyed, while others prefer to explore new styles and cultures, such as a European citizen desiring a North American prairie-style, Japanese or tropical garden. Irrespective of the style, the garden should be compatible with your principles and make sense to you in

Much of nature is driven by symmetry and systematic construction terms of its design. Gardens in which this isn't the case often feel inexplicably awkward.

For those who like symmetry or balance in their garden, there are many design features and plant options that can help. Regular, rectangular borders, patios and lawns can reflect the style of the surrounding architecture, and repetition of geometric shapes can be harmonious and provide consistency. Small trees such as *Cornus controversa* 'Variegata' (the wedding cake tree) and *C. alternifolia* (pagoda tree) have tiered branches that give strong horizontal lines, reflecting and reinforcing hard elements, such as fence tops and rooflines, and their common names very elegantly allude to this trait. A well-shaped, upright conifer provides a strong vertical dimension; a particular favourite of mine is the Korean fir (*Abies koreana*), with its strong lateral branches from which deep-purple cones push up at right angles, almost like toy soldiers on parade.

Symmetry also comes in circles. Look carefully at flowers and you will find that many are perfectly symmetrical. A ball *Dahlia* is archetypal of the perfect sphere, and a cactus *Dahlia* the exemplar intergalactic star. The arrangement of foliage fascinates, too. Species of *Sedum* and *Sempervivum* are composed of rosettes of overlapping triangular leaves that are almost hypnotic to peer into. These shapes can be used carefully to provide balance in the design, while also representing strong visual creativity.

Nature is ruled by geometry

Most of us think of nature as being composed of random elements: the unpredictability of a gust of wind perhaps, or the irregular appearance of primroses (*Primula vulgaris*) in a woodland. In reality, much of nature is driven by symmetry and systematic construction. Fractal shapes – shapes within shapes that repeat themselves at different scales – occur frequently in plants and other natural features. Fractals are perfectly formed symmetrical units and provide evidence that natural systems depend strongly on mathematical principles. Some psychologists think fractals are the reason we find natural features therapeutic, because the brain accepts these patterns and dimensions more readily than it does shapes that are less regular or coherent.

Health Benefit
Stress Reduction

Posited by Roger Ulrich in the 1980s, the Stress Reduction theory has some principles common to other key health theories, including Positive Affect, Attention Restoration and biophilia (see pages 62–3, 122–3 and 156–7). It suggests that positive emotions associated with viewing the natural world counteract negative thoughts and emotions, and by doing so inhibit psychophysiological stress. Viewing greenery, water, benign wildlife, beautiful flowers and so on causes a reduction in the body's physiological stress responses: the heart rate slows to normal, we breathe more easily and deeply, sweating is reduced, and there is a return to normal adrenalin and

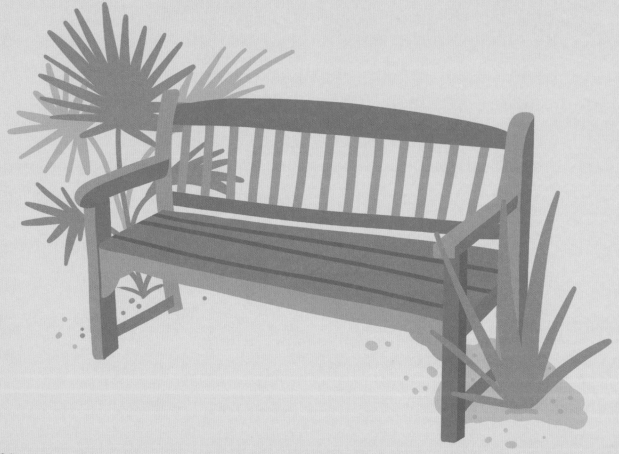

later cortisol (stress hormone) profiles.[8] There is also some evidence that people feel less pain or are able to tolerate pain better.[9]

The capacity to reduce stress through experiencing natural features is really important. It changes the arguments about how our cities should look, how citizens spend their working day, and even the activities people choose as recreation. Some government departments now recommend that everyone live within 300m (about 1,000ft) of a green space to provide them with a place to relax, and to help them cope better with the strains of modern life. While housing density is likely to increase to provide more homes, such residences must still offer high-quality green space. Inner-city locations without green space have been linked to higher stress, poorer mental health, more domestic violence and shorter lifespans. Some employers, too, now recognize that a de-stressed workforce is happier and more productive, and stays with the company longer. As a result, some are increasing the number of plants in and around their offices, and giving their employees opportunities to participate in lunchtime gardening clubs, park walks and so on.

Much of the evidence for stress relief relates to people viewing natural features, such as trees, parkland, flowers, fish swimming in a pool or grasses swaying in the breeze. But it is probably true that smelling certain aromas – particularly lavender and citronella – and hearing natural sounds, such as birdsong or whale 'music', also reduce adrenalin and other 'high-activation' responses associated with stress. Exposure to such stimuli can reduce stress in a matter of minutes, and regular bouts of 'natural relaxation' restore positive mood and regulate cortisol activity in the body. To capitalize on the benefits of these processes, though, we must remove ourselves from the adrenalin-inducing stimuli that are prevalent today – so the mobile phone ringtone should be muted and the email notifications silenced.

21 | Muse with Mood Boosters
Introduce majestic irises

The word 'iris' is linked with the ancient Greek term for a rainbow. This is very apt, since irises flower in every colour. They can be placed just about anywhere in the garden, and there are varieties suited to free-draining alpine beds and pots, hot baked-dry borders, shady woodland settings and even ponds. They are apt to bring a smile to your face (invoke positive affect) throughout the garden.

Perhaps the most spectacular are the bearded irises. These have broadsword-shaped leaves and tall flower stems that unfurl floral 'cloths' of gold, amber, cerise-pink and deepest inky blue, among many other colours, in early summer. Some are a single hue, while others boast one colour in the upper petals (standards) and a different colour in the lower (fall) petals. Irises are linked to royalty, and the flowers of the bearded irises are certainly regal. There are hundreds of different varieties, so it is worth searching out a specialist nursery. I find the 'black' varieties, such as 'Superstition', hugely dramatic, but I also use the red-browns (such as 'Dutch Chocolate') and tawnies (such as 'Patina') as conversation pieces. More 'conventional' blues (such as 'Blue Rhythm'), yellows (such as 'Minted Gold') and purples (such as 'Domination') remain the mainstays in my mixed borders. These bearded irises like their 'feet' (actually their rhizomes) to be baked in the sun, and do well against a warm, sunny wall. It's ideal to lift and divide them every three or four years to encourage them to keep flowering.

Another familiar iris is the one that is native to northern Europe: the yellow flag (*Iris pseudacorus*). This is commonly found growing at pond edges. It is the archetypal 'scaffolding' for dragonfly nymphs to climb up and escape their watery world. It is vigorous, though, so if you add it to your own water feature, you might want to confine it to a submerged basket. In North America, avoid this alien species entirely, and use instead the native *I. versicolor*, which naturally comes in a range of blue flowers.

Many people are introduced to irises by buying bulbs that send up their flowers in early spring. These are the dwarf iris: *Iris reticulata*, *I. histrioides* and similar 'alpine' or woodland species. Blue is the dominant colour, with varieties such as 'Katharine Hodgkin' and 'Frozen Planet' being the most fantastic pale electric-blue – a most unspringlike colour in many ways. Mix dwarf iris with *Crocus*, miniature *Narcissus* and early-flowering species tulips (*Tulipa*) in bowls and pots for superb colour early in the growing season. Once these plants finish flowering, simply place the bowls in a light but out-of-the-way corner, and let them rest up over the summer.

Finally, rather unheralded but great value are the Dutch and English irises (*Iris × hollandica*, and misleadingly named, since most of them originate from Spain and Portugal). These are large, bulbous irises. They do well in mixed borders, have fine, often veined flowers in blues, purples and yellow, and will multiply quietly from one year to the next.

The iris flower is so perfect that one can't help but admire it. It is a real bringer of joy, and although the individual flowers may not last very long, it is this fleeting perfection that creates such a wonderful emotion.

The iris flower is so perfect that one can't help but admire it

Memory Joggers
Use flower scents to stimulate the mind

22

Do you ever get a whiff of something and think, my goodness, that takes me back? One of the triggers for me is the sweet, lemony scent of some roses, which immediately carries me back to my aunt's garden on the east coast of Scotland, and warm summer holidays spent with cousins. I instantly picture the roses 'Blue Moon' and 'Chinatown' growing near her summerhouse. Despite originating in Scotland (which is not famous for its dry weather), the memories are positive and invariably the weather in them is sunny.

Some smells are immediately familiar and allow us to remember every moment, whereas in other situations the scent is transitory and the details of the memory elusive. These processes are not just a trick of the mind. Our sense of smell is processed by the limbic system of the brain, a component that also determines memory and, interestingly, emotions. Indeed, emotions are often integral to olfactory responses. Smells are not just linked to memory per se, but also potentially to feelings of nostalgia, love or remembrance. The perfume industry knows this very well, and scent is used to convey or elicit feelings of romance, relaxation, vitality and even power. Floral scents, such as rose, lavender and ylang-ylang, retain their popularity as perfumes.

So scent is a powerful mood enhancer. We can use this positively in the garden and around the house to take us away from the everyday, the mundane and the stressful. Flower perfumes can prompt positive memories or allow us to escape to times and places that made us happy. We might use the light, heavenly scent of honeysuckle (*Lonicera*) to escape to some fairy-tale woodland and imagine the sights and stirrings of the enchanted wood as we stroll through it on a cool summer's night. Alternatively, transport

Do roses manipulate us?

Plants developed perfumes (and floral colour) to attract pollinators. Some might argue that they are 'manipulating' insects to do their hard work for them in terms of spreading their genetic material (pollen) far and wide. The payment (a form of bribery, really) is a little drop of nectar. According to evolutionary theory, sex is fundamentally about an individual passing on their genes to the next generation and ideally expanding the range of the species through their progeny. For plants, the more seedlings they sire, the more successful the individual and, indeed, the species.

So pollinators are unwittingly helping these plant species in their attempts at botanical world domination. But then there is another species that propagates and spreads plants by the million around the globe: humans. At least with crop plants, humans get some benefit too – we can eat them. But what substantive benefit do we get from growing a rose? Is it possible that roses and other flowering plants are manipulating us? We have spread these plants around the world, and, in evolutionary terms, the rose family, Rosaceae, must be considered one of the most successful. Why? Because they simply look good and smell wonderful. Some researchers have suggested that, unlike other gifts we give to family or lovers, plants and flowers have no evolutionary or material benefit. These plants are acting on our emotions alone. It's just a thought, but next time you plant a rose, consider who is exploiting whom.

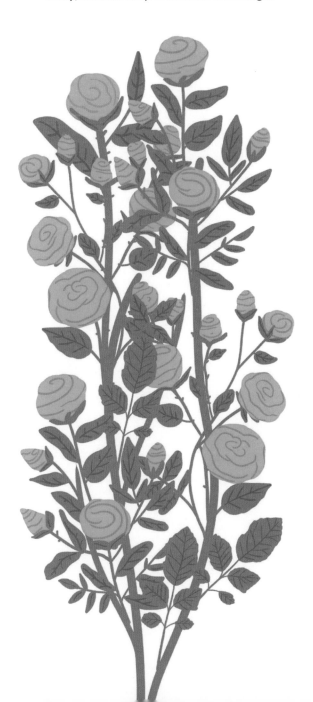

Some scents are immediately familiar and allow us to remember every moment, whereas in other situations the scent is transitory and the details of the memory elusive

Winter wonders

In the cool, short days of winter, flowering plants draw in the few pollinating insects around (usually small flies and midges) with strong scent. They include wintersweet (*Chimonanthus praecox*), sweet box (*Sarcococca confusa*), the spiky, architectural form that is Oregon grape (*Mahonia*) and (in my opinion) the most fabulous of them all: the *Daphne* species and cultivars. *Daphne* has a reputation for being fickle, growing nicely for many years and then suddenly collapsing and dying. But these plants really are worth the effort, despite this. I am not aware of any other plant that brings a whole garden alive simply by its wonderful, majestic aroma. The flowers, which are small and tend to be white, pale purple or yellow (depending on the species), are attractive in themselves, albeit on a demure, subtle scale. But they pack a punch when it comes to making their presence felt through scent. Given a still, warmish sunny day in late winter, these sirens of scent can captivate from 50m (165ft) or more away.

yourself to the Far East with the intoxicating scent of jasmines (such as *Jasminum officinale* and *J. polyanthum*) and roses (such as *Rosa banksiae* 'Lutescens'). Reawaken memories of Mediterranean holidays with lavender (*Lavandula*), sage (*Salvia officinalis*) and coronilla (*Coronilla valentina* subsp. *glauca*). Or use scent to relax and rejuvenate. Where the summers are warm, grow *Citrus* (oranges, grapefruit, lemons and limes) to provide soothing aroma, and where the weather is not consistently warm (are we back in Scotland?), try the 'mock' alternatives *Philadelphus* and *Choisya ternata*, which have equally evocative scents.

My team and I are interested in the extent to which flower scent affects human well-being. My colleague Dr Lauriane Chalmin-Pui has carried out a number of experiments at the Royal Horticultural Society's Garden Wisley in Surrey, United Kingdom, to determine how floral scent affects people's emotions, and whether some scents are better than others at promoting positive or relaxing moods.

Scent is a
powerful mood
enhancer

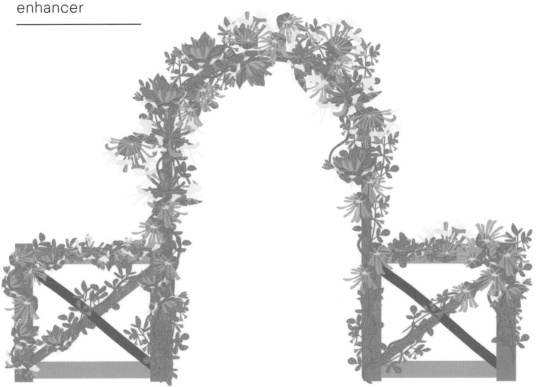

Honeysuckle by the gate

Honeysuckle (*Lonicera periclymenum*) is a
paradigm of the English cottage garden,
a style often associated with charm and
antiquity. It is native to northwestern Europe
and grows in woodland, so it didn't take
much effort to transplant it to a place by
many a British front door or garden gate.
Real cottage gardeners were nothing if not
utilitarian – 'adapt' and 'make do' being the
watchwords – and useful and colourful wild
plants 'jumped over' the hedge to take pride
of place in the garden. You can use the native
form of this plant to transport yourself back
to this simpler world, but cultivars such as
'Serotina' (with larger, red-backed flowers)

and 'Graham Thomas' (more delicate
yellow-and-cream flowers) are worth
considering too. Place your chosen plant
where it will release its scent as you brush
past it. Watch out, on balmy evenings, as
honeysuckles try to catch the attention
of their favourite pollinators, and you
might hear the drone of the spectacular
elephant hawkmoth doing its rounds of the
flowers. In North America, the native coral
honeysuckle (*L. sempervirens*) may be a
better choice; it will attract ruby-throated
hummingbirds, as well as supporting the
caterpillars of spring azure butterflies and
snowberry clearwing moths.

23 | The Myriad Life
Keep ornamental plants in the home

Plants lend a softening, reassuring feel to our living spaces

Our most intimate spaces are within our homes. If we tolerate the presence here of life forms other than our own, that is a good sign that we have a strong connection to nature. Indeed, for many, the simple houseplant is the single closest connection to the natural environment. Plants, in turn, repay this 'trust' of cohabitation by providing interest and distraction from the strain of everyday life. Some of the earliest studies associated with biophilic responses involved plants inside buildings, not outside. This research showed that interior planting reduced stress, increased pain tolerance, improved productivity in offices and enhanced the academic performance of students, mostly through increasing their attention span.

Plants lend a softening, reassuring feel to our living spaces. They soften the hard edges of interior decor and remove the impression of sterility. Interior designers (and most homeowners) recognize this, and frequently exploit plants for the atmosphere they bring. But plants can also – through cultural associations – reinforce design styles and the impressions conveyed by other decorative elements. If we desire an Edwardian-styled dining room, wicker furniture, curved lamps and pale, clean paint schemes are essential, but so are parlour palms (*Chamaedorea elegans*), with their elegant dissected leaves. The open structure of the furniture is further matched by silhouettes of *Ficus benjamina* 'Twilight', with its gently sweeping branches, and foxtail ferns (*Asparagus densiflorus* 'Myersii'). If you prefer a 'clean-living' style with slate floors, white panelling, Cubist couches and modern art on the walls, seek bold plant forms. Strong architectural shapes are supplied by *Philodendron*, *Ficus elastica*, *Spathiphyllum* 'Alana' and *Sansevieria cylindrica*, the last with rocket-like stems that erupt skywards.

Bathroom cabinets and windowsills are ideal for trailing plants such as the wandering sailor (*Tradescantia*), of which the variety 'Sweetness' has trailing stems with green, white and mauve-flushed leaves. The classic easy-to-grow bathroom specimen is the spider plant (*Chlorophytum comosum*). It comes most commonly in variegated forms (those with green-and-white leaves), but I like 'Lemon', with its fresh, grass-like colouring. Both these plants are easy to propagate from stem cuttings, or from natural offshoots (baby plants) in the case of *Chlorophytum* – so share them with friends.

For flowers, consider African violets or Cape primroses (both now classified as *Steptocarpus*, although many people still recall African violets as *Saintpaulia*). The latter come in a range of heavenly blues and purples, as well as reds, pinks and white. The flowers of Cape primroses are on a more noticeable short stalk, and often have a distinctively coloured 'throat' in the centre. These also come in a great selection of colours, and include speckled and bicoloured flowers. African violets and Cape primroses both resent hot, direct sunlight, so diffuse light or an east- or north-facing windowsill (south-facing in the southern hemisphere) suits them best.

Pet-friendly?

Cats and dogs have a tendency to chew things, so take care that your furry and leafy friends are compatible. Some houseplants are toxic (including *Spathiphyllum*, *Dieffenbachia*, *Strelitzia*, *Aloe* and *Philodendron*), so be sure to have all the facts before leaving your pet unattended in the house.

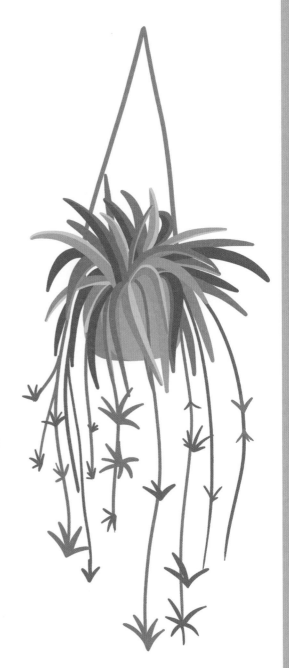

24 Grasp the Green Sponge
Design and build a rain garden

Viewing vegetation and feeling relaxed or more positive about life is sometimes called green therapy. Being around and viewing water, or even being involved in watersports, such as swimming, canoeing and surfing, is often referred to as blue therapy, thanks to the mental-health boost associated with such activities.

Where the blue element is definitely not therapeutic, though, is when it threatens to engulf your property or affect your livelihood – namely through flooding. Flooding, along with other dangerous phenomena, such as fire, drought and wind damage, is on the increase because of climate change. All these are distinct and increasing sources of anxiety for many people. But one way to reduce the risk of urban flooding is to adopt SuDS – sustainable urban drainage systems. SuDS use the 'lie of the land' and vegetation to hold back and store rainwater. One of the most important things we can do as individuals to contribute to the reduction of local flooding is to build a rain garden. A network of rain gardens and similar swales (moist, low-lying areas) introduced across our towns and cities can combine to act as a significant reservoir for rainwater. What's more, by creating a rain garden you will make your own little blue/green therapeutic haven. Two benefits for the price of one!

A rain garden is effectively a shallow scoop in the ground, where the base has been dug out and backfilled with a free-draining substrate that helps water to drain into the ground. A pipe (or, if you prefer, a rill; see chapter 49) is run from a nearby downpipe (downspout) on a building so that rainwater from the roof enters the rain garden rather than going into the land drain or sewage system. But this is not just a *bare* scoop in the ground; plants are added to turn it into a unique garden feature. Most rain gardens feature ornamental plants

By creating a rain garden you will make your own little blue/green therapeutic haven

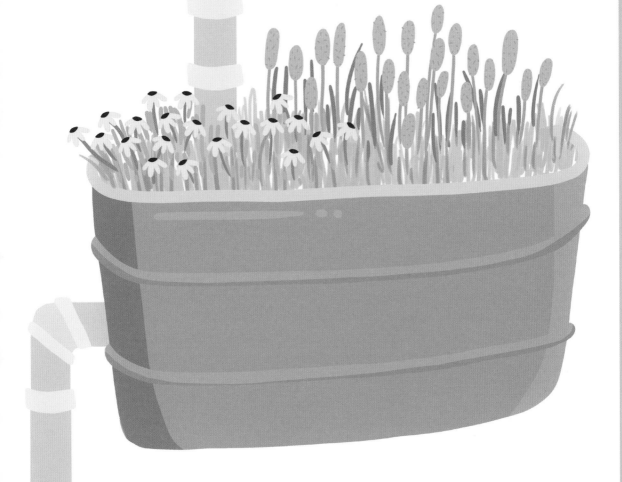

or less vigorous native species that make the garden look attractive and enticing to relax in.

Rain gardens are not consistently wet. During rain-free periods they may dry out, starting from the upper edges of the depression and finishing with the centre. And this gradient is ecologically interesting. Some plants like the predominately wet centre, while others prefer the edge of the depression, which tends to be drier and more free-draining. For the damp centre, choose striking plants, such as the globe flower (*Trollius × cultorum* 'Orange Princess') or cardinal flower (*Lobelia cardinalis* 'Queen Victoria'). A little further out from the centre, use daylilies (*Hemerocallis*), with their bold masses of yellow, orange, scarlet or pink flowers, or *Astilbe*, with its feather-duster flowers in red, white or pink. At the upper edges of the scoop you might include tufted hair grass (*Deschampsia cespitosa*) for its flowing movement, and perhaps speedwells (*Veronica*) and catmint (*Nepeta*), with their restful panicles in blues and mauves. Animal life will follow, with various amphibians loving the damp centre and the shady conditions provided by the plants. Watch out, too, for the tiny pollen beetle, *Meligethes aeneus*, like a scattering of black beads on the yellow flowers of *Hemerocallis*.

Plants that like wet conditions are often exuberant in their growth, because of the simple fact that water is rarely a limiting factor. Some of the most pernicious and rampant weeds are associated with

Stormwater planter

This form of mini rain garden is another useful SuDS intervention. It is much smaller – the rain-garden equivalent of a window box – and could brighten up an alley at the side of the house, or be a colourful feature on the facade of a domestic building. It consists of a metal or plastic tank, part of which is designed to hold rainwater after a heavy storm. The building's downpipe is the input, but the overflow outlet pipe can be set at different levels; the higher up it is, the wetter the system will be, and the greater its capacity for water storage. A lower output point will mean a drier system. Either way, there are plants to suit your chosen regime, with rushes and reeds at the wet end of the spectrum and perhaps 'self-watering' tomatoes (*Lycopersicon esculentum*) and cabbages (*Brassica oleracea*) at the drier end.

The green oasis in the urban block

A well-designed rain garden will provide plenty of restoration for the soul, not least because water run-off is often problematic in incongruous places, such as alongside roads, in community housing schemes or by apartments. A little green oasis in such places provides respite from the strains of working life, commuting or neighbourhood tension. Adding a little colour or attracting wildlife will improve spirits and bring a feeling of balance for those who live nearby. So much the better if this mini-landscape can be managed by the community, thereby providing opportunities for social engagement and making new friends.

the banks of rivers and other waterways, especially if non-native, competitive species manage to get a foothold there. Such species – among them Himalayan balsam (*Impatiens glandulifera*) in western Europe and purple loosestrife (*Lythrum salicaria*) in North America – can rapidly crowd out the native plants. So, for the wetter parts of the rain garden, it is wise to consider species that are not too aggressive in their growth habit, and to be prepared to cut back and thin out the vegetation from time to time.

With time, leaf litter and the natural aggregation of soil particles rolling down the slopes of the rain garden may result in a thick layer of rich, oozy mud at the base. Scooping out this excess silt every two or three years will help to keep the rain garden functional. Be sure to leave the residue at the top edge of the rain garden for a week or so (as you would if cleaning a pond), to allow any stranded amphibians or moisture-loving invertebrates to crawl back down to the damper areas.

Health Benefit
Physical Activity

Physical movement is vitally important to us. The 'well-oiled' machine that is the human body must be run regularly to keep it in good shape. About 33 per cent of adults worldwide do not do enough physical exercise. In the United States, sedentary behaviour (desk work, watching TV, playing video games and so on) typically accounts for about eight hours of daytime activity. This inactivity is a major problem and underpins many health difficulties. Indeed, physical inactivity is the fourth most common cause of premature death, and the cause of numerous preventable physical and mental disorders.

At a biochemical level, a sedentary lifestyle reduces lipoprotein lipase activity, protein transport and carbohydrate metabolism, and impairs lipid (fat) metabolism and the circulation of sex hormones. These factors then affect physiological processes, resulting in a greater likelihood of heart disease, diabetes, cancers (such as bowel, breast and prostate), dementia and a plethora of mental-health problems. In the United Kingdom, for example, if

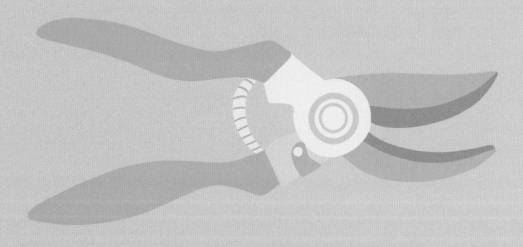

people were to increase their physical activity by just 10 per cent, the health services would save £500 million and life would be prolonged for 6,000 citizens every year.

It is clear that the modern lifestyle means humans must find feasible ways of exercising more. Gardening is a great way to exercise regularly. Activities such as pushing a lawnmower, vigorously raking leaves or digging the soil burn 400 calories an hour, as well as improving cardiovascular performance, muscle strength and dexterity, and strengthening bones.[10] Gardening is considered useful in reducing the likelihood of osteoporosis in later life, and it has been shown to be more effective than walking, self-education activities or moderate alcohol consumption in protecting against dementia. Thus, it also has implications for mental health, as it keeps the mind active, enhances self-esteem and can aid social connections. It is often (although not always) inexpensive and is therefore a useful activity for retired people or those on tight budgets.

One great advantage of gardening, along with a number of other eco-therapies, is that it is addictive. If you are a keen gardener, you don't need motivation to be out there potting, weeding, planting and enjoying the colours and shapes you have created. Gardening encourages regular activity, and frequent, short bouts of movement are very effective at keeping the human engine in good condition. Studies on patients recovering from stroke or heart attack have found that exercise in a garden was more effective, enjoyable and sustainable than therapy in traditional, formal recuperation settings.

Gardening seems to encourage physical activity in the long term, and not be a flash-in-the-pan phenomenon, in contrast to so many New Year's resolutions about going to the gym. Overdo it, of course, and you may encounter problems. Gardeners often suffer back or joint pain, but that is generally because they have done it for hours nonstop. Gardening should be a series of light 'warm-ups', not marathons, and to that end I find interspersing cups of tea with the planting and pruning an attractive strategy.

25 | **Pushing Power**
Invest in a push lawnmower

As a rule, humans like their landscapes to be about one third upright structure and two thirds open plain. Many gardeners like a bit of lawn as that open plain, valuing the space and freedom of movement it brings to the garden. A grass lawn is the ideal open plain, and highly functional at that. It stops the garden from becoming congested; it is the platform from which we can view all our 'plant performers'; it allows us to stroll past the flower borders or partake in a game of football with the kids; and it offers space for the dog, rabbit or chickens to romp around.

Mowing the lawn manually can burn about 300–400 calories an hour, and improves cardiovascular function

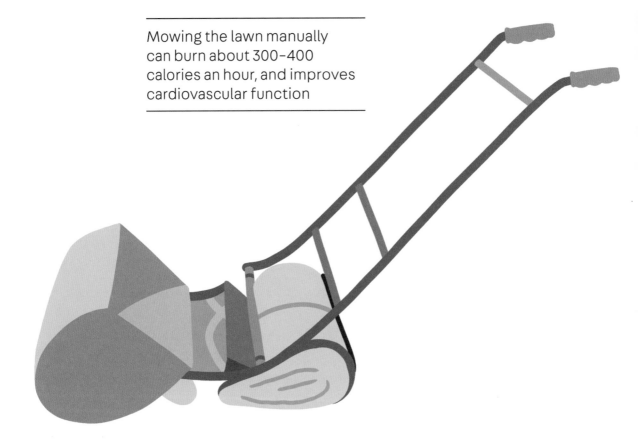

Having said that, in the gardening world there is nothing so controversial as the lawn. If you want a lawn that looks immaculate, like Centre Court at Wimbledon, be prepared to throw amazing amounts of labour, energy, water and fertilizer at it. At the other end of the spectrum there is plastic grass; it will give you a carefree lawn, but at what cost to Mother Nature? Nothing lives in or under plastic.

Neither of these options is good for the environment, but there is a much more benign middle way. This is to manage a lawn in a sustainable manner, not be too worried about the occasional daisy or buttercup, and let the grasses adapt to the weather and the degree of wear and tear you impose on them. Lawn grasses are amazingly resilient and will bounce back after periods of drought (when they can look somewhat brown) or when someone has pitched a tent on them for three weeks and they turn an insipid yellow. The key aims with this third way are for the lawn to survive, to provide habitat for insects and other invertebrates, and even to improve your own physical health.

Mowing the lawn about once every two weeks will keep it manageable. (Leave the grass to grow too long and you will need to resort to a strimmer or scythe; see page 102.) A manual cylinder push-mower will give you the best exercise, and is also a quieter

Meadow magic

If you have a reasonably large lawn, you could leave some areas uncut for longer to create more plant diversity and provide food and shelter for minibeasts. Leave these areas for between six and ten weeks, to let the grass grow to about 10–15cm (4–6in) high. The longer grass allows low-growing wild flowers to put in an appearance. Some people leave most of the lawn like this and cut paths through only in the direction of destinations they wish to access, such as the shed, the washing line or the patio. Others prefer most of the lawn to be the traditional close-mown sward, and to leave rougher patches as swathes within it. You can even make attractive shapes such as swirls, circles or Paisley patterns, to be seen from above.

When it comes to cutting these wilder areas again, you will need to lift the blade height of a conventional mower for the first cut, then lower it for a second cut. Alternatively, use a strimmer to cut back longer grass.

option. Most have a set of wheels, a cylinder composed of curved blades and another flat blade at the base, and a handle for you to push against. The blades work in tandem to give the grass a neat, sharp cut, just like nail scissors. Mowing the lawn manually can burn about 300–400 calories an hour, and improves cardiovascular function. Physical exertion of this kind, where the heart rate increases above 50 per cent of its capacity continuously for 20–30 minutes, improves physical fitness. As such, mowing is in effect an outdoor workout, like cycling or jogging – and, what's more, you are creating a fine green veneer for the garden at the same time.

If you don't fancy the full physical workout, electric mowers (and other garden equipment) are available, and still involve a degree of physical exercise. Ideally, powered machinery should use rechargeable batteries and a green source of energy from the grid to minimize carbon emissions.

Should you let the grass grow really long, as was traditionally done in hay, riverside or alpine meadows, the scythe is the tool of choice for cutting the hay effectively. Using a scythe is an art, and even after ten years I'm not sure I have perfected it. You can go on a course to improve your sweep and angle of cut, and a very sharp blade tends to help too. Even if you don't perfect it, scything is still very useful exercise for the hips and stomach. I manage most of my grass as meadow, and although that means that four or five weekends

What is in the magic mix?

Wild-flower species will be able to colonize longer areas of grass in a meadow. Depending on soil type, climate and frequency of cutting, you may find adventurers such as daisy (*Bellis perennis*), slender speedwell (*Veronica filiformis*), white clover (*Trifolium repens*), red clover (*T. pratense*), fox and cubs (*Pilosella aurantiaca*) and even the occasional meadow orchid (such as *Dactylorhiza*). If you are lucky enough to get orchids, do not mow the meadow, but let the plants die back naturally. Areas of temporary no-mow grass are also useful for letting the foliage of spring bulbs, such as snowdrops (*Galanthus*), *Crocus* and tulips (*Tulipa*), die back gracefully. Apeldoorn tulips, being robust, are especially good in grass.

around midsummer are dominated by scything, I find the result very satisfying. I always balance the hard work with significant rest periods in a deckchair.

Ideally, after cutting hay, keep the grass short for the rest of the summer by going back to the manual mower. This job is done for me by my pet geese, which are released to graze on the meadow. I don't recommend this solution for everyone, especially those in towns, since geese can be noisy and the ganders are rather aggressive during the breeding season – but some might say that being pursued regularly by belligerent geese is another useful way of keeping fit.

Other physical workouts

Mowing the lawn is probably the most regular form of physical exercise in the garden, but weeding with a hoe, turning over the compost heap and trimming a hedge with hand shears are also useful for keeping you toned up and supple. Heavy lifting is often a requirement, too, but do be careful not to overstrain the body. Supporting the back and bending at the knees are important to avoid back injury.

26 Rapid Greening
Germinate edible nasturtiums

Nasturtiums (*Tropaeolum majus*) are little bonfires of colour, their trumpet flowers ablaze with flaming orange, deep scarlet, velvety red and breezy yellow. They will brighten odd corners in the garden and quickly screen unsightly sheds or garage walls. The natural form is a climber that grows to 2–3m (6–10ft) in height, but there are now dwarf varieties that you can easily accommodate in hanging baskets and window boxes. Recent varieties have also widened the colour spectrum to off-pink and palest lemon. Where I grew up, nasturtiums were called 'nippy biscuits', the leaves being edible and tasting a bit like peppermint with an extra kick. The leaf shape itself is interesting, having a central point attached to the stem and radiating veins holding the off-circular leaf section in place, a bit like a lopsided cartwheel.

Very few plants are as easy to germinate and grow as the nasturtium; indeed, it is more difficult to spell the name than it is to grow the plant. The pea-sized seeds are readily poked into the soil in late spring, after all danger of frost has passed. These are very forgiving plants and actually flower best on poor soil, so they can be popped into those spare pockets of earth that are often found around the base of the house walls. If you are relaxed about gardening (and surely that is what this book is trying to encourage), they will self-seed around over subsequent years, finding sheltered places so as to avoid being killed by frost.

Ease of cultivation, rapid growth, vibrant flower colour and the fact that the leaves and flowers are edible make nasturtiums a firm favourite with children, and really fun to grow. Such activities are important for the child, not only in social and bonding terms, but also as a doorway to better engagement with nature and discovering the fun of growing plants. These pursuits are important for mental and social development, but scientists also believe that exposure to the natural environment during the formative years boosts and trains the immune system (see pages 136–7). Children are *designed* to jump in puddles and play in the mud. It's natural and, contrary to popular belief, it probably reduces the risk of disease and infection over the long term, compared to keeping children in semi-sealed, 'sterile' environments. So encourage your children to ramble through the garden and poke seeds into the mud – and nasturtiums are a rewarding place to start.

The fact that
the leaves and
flowers are
edible makes
nasturtiums
a firm favourite
with children

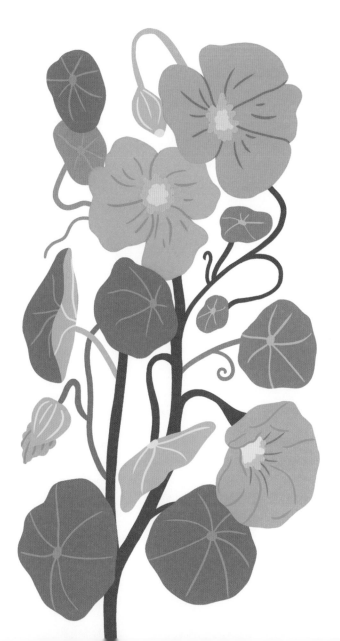

27 | **Berry Bonanza**
Colour your fall with beautiful berries

Autumn is a great time for colour and atmosphere. Many people love the red, gold and auburn 'fireworks' we experience as the leaves change hue and the nights grow chillier. But remember that autumn is not just about leaf colour, but also the season of 'mists and mellow fruitfulness'. It is harvesting and fruiting time. Trees and shrubs become festooned with berries, nuts and colourful little apples, which can themselves be surprisingly bright.

There are many small trees that will suit even the most limited garden, and the rowans or mountain ash (*Sorbus*) are among the most spectacular in autumn. The berries of some contrast dramatically with the turning foliage, such as *S.* 'Joseph Rock', with bright-yellow berries against a backdrop of purple-red leaves that are truly spectacular in low autumn sunlight. *S. pseudohupehensis* 'Pink Pagoda' is wreathed in pink berries in late autumn, before the berries fade to a wintry white. The ornamental crab apples (*Malus*) provide variety in terms of both fruit size and colour. *M. hupehensis* has cherry-sized fruit, whereas *M.* 'Wisley Crab' has distinctive deep-maroon fruit the size of a dessert apple. If yellow or gold is your colour, look for *M.* 'Butterbur', 'Golden Hornet' and 'Golden Gem'. All the ornamental *Malus* have the bonus of lovely spring blossom.

Where space is precious, shrubs are more appropriate. The *Cotoneaster* species and cultivars come mostly with small but numerous red or orange berries. One notable exception is *C. rothschildianus*,

Regulating the body

Maintaining an interest in the outdoors throughout the year is important for both physical and mental health. Seasonal effects and light levels help to set our body clock and improve sleep patterns, and we need sunlight to produce vitamin D, especially in the winter. Spending time outdoors may be particularly important for children, to encourage physical development and mental resilience.

Plants that maintain interest
through autumn and into winter
may even produce the strongest
and most spectacular colours of
the entire year

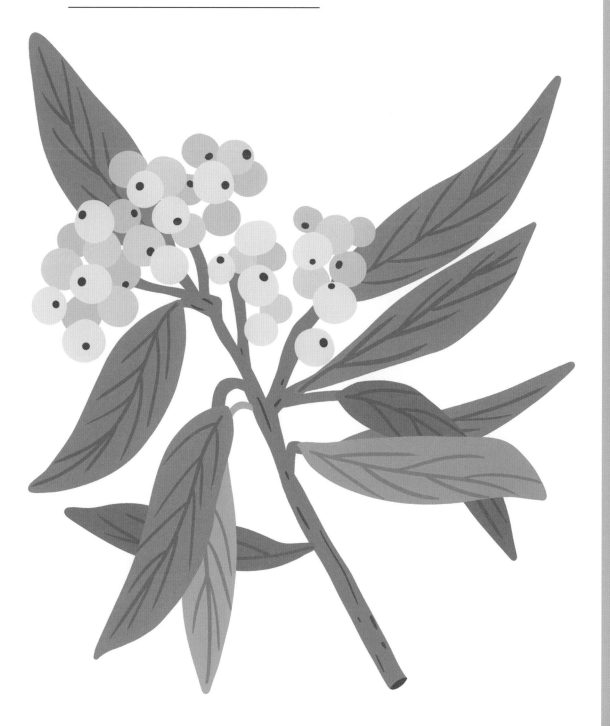

Strong colours are important
in keeping us interested in our
gardens, parks and other outdoor
spaces as the days grow cooler

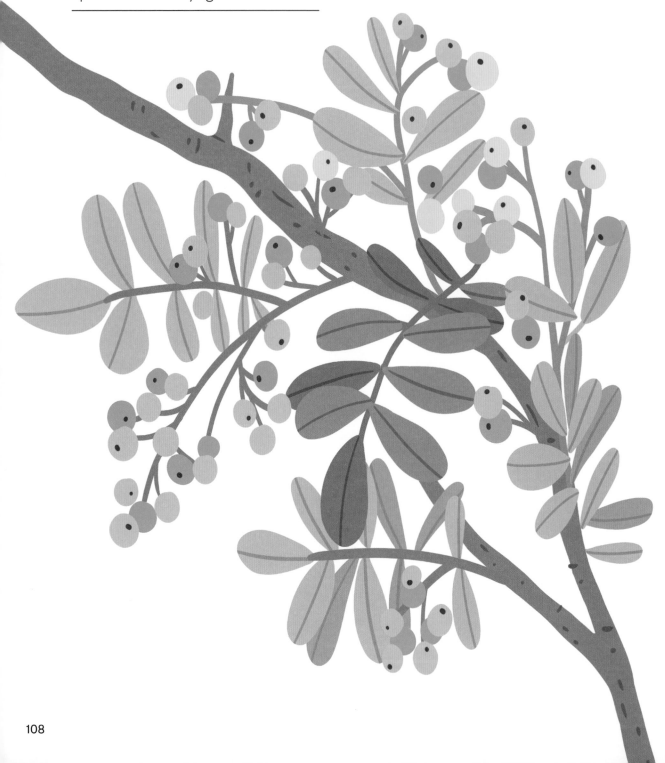

with its pale-sulphur-coloured fruit, a lovely match to its mid-green foliage, which it retains throughout the winter. For bright, almost fluorescent purple, go for *Callicarpa bodinieri* var. *giraldii* 'Profusion'; its berries are like a laser beam on the retina, and it's no wonder this shrub has picked up the common name 'beautyberry'. Not as spectacular, but also an unusual colour, are the deep-blue berries of *Viburnum davidii*, a plant that has other attractions, with its flattened heads of white flowers and its elliptical, strongly veined leaves of deep green. *V. lantana* produces eye-catching clusters of both black and red berries together. Finally, another *Viburnum* I would squeeze in is guelder rose (*V. opulus*), with scarlet berries that keep the birds fed over winter.

All these strong colours are important in keeping us interested in our gardens, parks and other outdoor spaces as the days grow cooler and the days shorter. It is thought that gardeners do 50–75 per cent less physical work during winter than in summer, so anything that prolongs our interest in the outdoors and stops us from becoming too sedentary is a good thing. As a bonus, plants that maintain interest through autumn and into winter may even produce the strongest and most spectacular colours of the entire year.

Nature deficit disorder

For those who grew up without computers and mobile phones (essentially the Dark Ages, according to my students), playing outdoors was as natural as falling off a log. That is not true today, when children may spend up to eight hours a day sitting in front of some kind of screen, despite two hours being the maximum recommended. Their capacity to explore the neighbourhood and wider natural spaces is reined in by concerns over traffic and the fear of abduction.

But such social changes have ramifications for health and the environment. Spending more time outdoors is linked with greater physical fitness and a lower body mass index in children. Children who do not engage with the natural world (so-called nature deficit disorder) are less likely to be concerned about the degradation of the environment, including key issues such as climate change. One of the very few positives to come out of the COVID-19 pandemic was greater numbers of children appreciating their gardens and local parks; some even went so far as to take up gardening.

Health Benefit
Thermal Comfort

Our bodies are designed to run efficiently at a core temperature of
35–37.5°C (95–99.5°F). They are constantly reacting to the external
environment to maintain this temperature by 'burning' calories
(that is to say, using energy from food) in cold environments to keep
us warm, and perspiring in warm environments to ensure that we
remain cool. What we experience on the outside (skin temperature)
is temperature in relation to our own thermal comfort zone. This
is subjective, and depends on genetics, climate (including relative
humidity and wind speed), metabolic rate (how fast the individual
can use calories), clothing and physical movement.

Heat stress is a killer, and excessive temperature can injure the
brain and other vital organs. Climate change is warming the
planet in such a way as to make the hot places hotter, but also the
cool places exceptionally warm at times. In the latter parts of the
world the population is not used to or adapted to extreme heat.
The heatwave in central Europe in 2003, for example, caused an
extra 15,000 fatalities, and the elderly, the very young and those
with heart or respiratory problems suffered most. This is a vicious
circle in environmental terms, too. It is predicted that by 2060 more
energy will be used globally to cool buildings than to warm them
– a sobering thought when you consider that humans invented
houses to keep them warm and dry.

Plants keep us cool. The fact that they shade building exteriors
makes trees, climbing plants and green roofs a notable form of
passive cooling, helping to dissipate the solar energy that makes
our houses and offices so warm in summer. Outdoor cooling is also
important in some climates. It's no accident that village elders
meet under the thorn acacias of Kenya and Tanzania to discuss

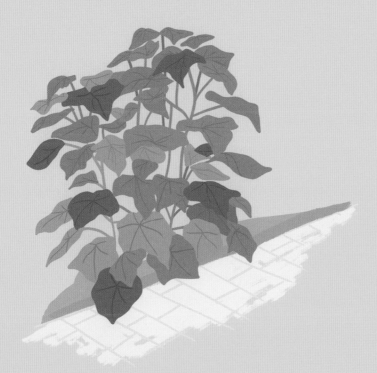

village politics, or that French Riviera society congregates around café tables in the shade of large trees. Plants also act as natural air-conditioning units.[11] They use sunlight to turn liquid water into vapour, and it is this change of state in water that dissipates solar energy, thus avoiding further increases in the surrounding air temperature.

On a hot summer's day green (and blue) spaces are distinctly cooler. The air temperature in a park on the warmest day might be 2–3ºC (3–6°F) cooler, and in the countryside 8–10ºC (14–18°F) cooler, than in the city centre. In hot climates the presence of trees by buildings reduces the energy required for air conditioning by 30–50 per cent. In temperate countries similar planting can eliminate the need for artificial air conditioning completely, by keeping a building interior below 24ºC (75°F) through passive cooling alone. Even in cities in temperate climates, where a lack of adaptation to heat is a problem, trees prove useful. In research my students conducted in Sheffield, northern England, street trees cooled pavements and roads consistently by a tangible 5ºC (9°F) on uncomfortably hot afternoons.[12]

28 Great and Small Green Walls
Create a mini green wall in your backyard

I have always been spellbound by where plants grow. Playing among the rocks on the beach as a child, I would sometimes be stopped short by a face-to-face encounter with a plant that seemed to be growing directly out of the rock. I was dumbfounded then, and still am today, by the way a plant such as thrift (*Armeria maritima*) can hang on in such an inhospitable environment. Not only does it survive, but also, when in flower, it looks opulent and stunning. Its

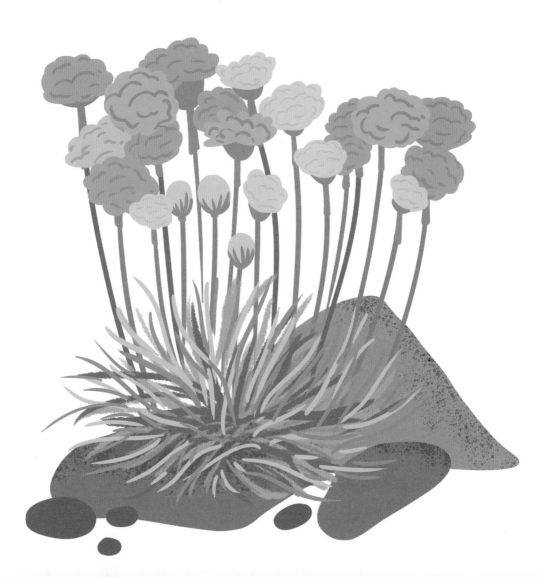

tenacity is not to be underestimated, with its small pink pompom flowers flying in the face of briny blasts from the sea. I went on to study for a Ph.D in how plants adapt to their environments, but that simple captivation with plants' survival against the odds has never left me. Such moments of captivation can be highly distracting, and provide the brain with downtime from everyday worries.

Replicating a coastal cliff around your house or in your garden might not be feasible, but you can create similar conditions, and be equally astonished by the way plants adapt and grow. Green or living walls have become popular in commercial settings since the turn of the millennium, and are often used by companies to suggest 'green' (environmental) credentials, even when they don't really have any. Such green walls are usually large and complex, but you can do something much smaller, simpler and more intimate. If you want luxuriant plants hanging free and screening a fence or wall, choose a module or container system, which you can water easily by hand or via drip-irrigation tubing. Even better, make this system more sustainable by linking it to the guttering and letting the rain provide the irrigation. Such green screens readily accommodate plants of the type that suit hanging baskets, and can include trailing *Fuchsia*, *Begonia* and *Lobelia*, as well as the hardworking *Diascia*, *Nemesia* and *Verbena*, which are in constant flower throughout the summer.

Personally, I like the plant communities that don't rely on us for constant watering. These include the true alpines and succulents, tough plants that are designed to hang on and survive despite the adverse conditions that nature throws at them. They are specialists in drought, wind, cold and even sometimes heat. Interestingly, such species will not last five minutes if they are asked to compete with more vigorous plants in a community, such as in a meadow. They actually need sparse, rocky, nutrient-poor, wind-blown conditions if they are to do well.

For such plants, a great solution is to build small green walls – about 1.5m (4–5ft) high at most, using engineering bricks in a double layer.

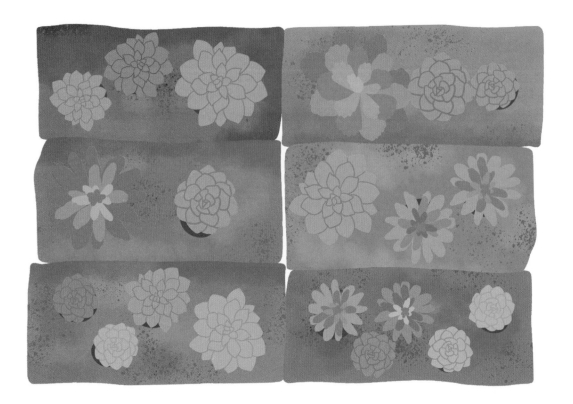

You will be
astonished
by the way
plants adapt
and grow

These are the bricks with three holes, intentionally designed – or so it seems – for popping an alpine plant into. Key to such a feature is that the wall be open at the top so rainwater can get in from above. The infill between the two brick 'skins' is a sandy aggregate mixed with organic matter, such as garden compost, to provide some nutrition and aid moisture retention. Similar brick structures can be built as retaining walls where the ground changes level naturally. In this case, moisture can get in from the back (the side that abuts the soil), so the wall does not need to be open at the top. Either way, use the bricks with the holes facing out to create mini-caves into which plants can be squeezed.

When planting an alpine or succulent plant in such a 'cave', it is important that the roots make good contact with the substrate at the back of the brick, because they need access to the water within it if they are to get themselves established. Such spots are ideal for saxifrages (*Saxifraga*), the epitome of alpine toughness.

There are the mossy types, with their soft green leaves and tiny lamp-post-shaped flowers, which provide a great contrast to the hardness of the wall. They flower in shades of pink, red or white, and common varieties include 'Peter Pan' and 'Pixie'. 'Cloth of Gold' is a gold-leaved form best put in shade to show off its colour and avoid scorching. In contrast to the mossy types, the semi-spherical cushion saxifrages are almost as hard as stone (they may look like a cushion, but not one you would want to sit on). Some are silver saxifrages, so called because of the white-blue deposits on the leaves; this is encrusted limestone (calcium carbonate), adding to the stony appearance. The cushions, which are already a fantastic shape, really come into their own when these tight mounds have a halo of pink, white or yellow flowers.

Other slots in a green wall can accommodate *Aubretia*, which is available in lavender, blue and pink forms. These make wonderful 'living waterfalls' tumbling down the face of the brickwork. To provide a stark contrast, consider the acid yellows of gold dust (*Aurinia saxatilis*) or golden alyssum (*Alyssum saxatile*). For hotter, drier spots, houseleeks (*Sempervivum*) and stonecrops (*Sedum*) are the plants of choice, with their fleshy, drought-resistant leaves in green, red or purple. Don't forget the top of the wall – it's a good location for dwarf *Dianthus*, alpine phlox (*Phlox subulata* and *P. douglasii*) and rock roses (*Helianthemum*).

Green walls on show

I designed an exhibit at the RHS Chelsea Flower Show in 2010 to demonstrate the role of green walls. I constructed two walls that were mirror images of each other, but one was planted and one was not. An infrared camera showed the temperature of each. The planted wall was about 8°C (just over 14°F) cooler, clearly demonstrating plants' potential for cooling buildings. This kind of engagement with the public is really important in demonstrating the role science plays in trying to find solutions to everyday problems, and this particular exhibit illustrated that garden plants are not only attractive, but also can be highly functional.

29 | **Cheeky Faces**
Plant cheery pansies and violas

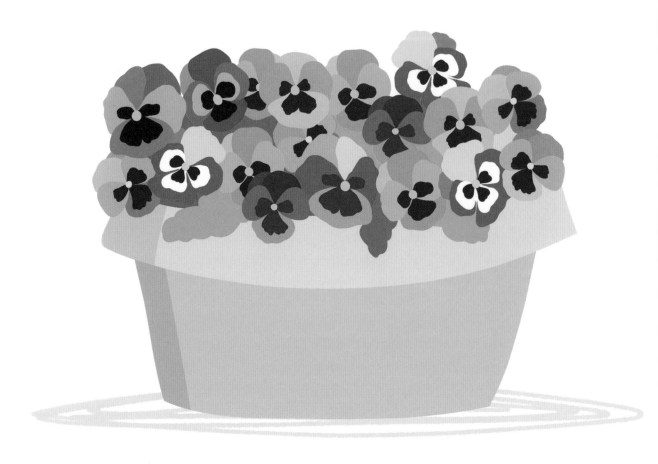

Even better the second time around

Pansies and violas are members of the violet
family, and their wild ancestor still grows
on field margins in sandy soils. Collect
seed from your own plants at the end of the
flowering season, keep them dry over winter,
and sow them in free-draining compost on
a windowsill in spring. When they are 6–10cm

(2–4in) tall, plant them out into troughs
or pots. These plants cross-fertilize each
other, so a whole range of unique and
unexpected flower colours will arise in
every seed-sown generation. They are
always a source of surprise and wonder.

The familiar pansy and viola (*Viola × wittrockiana*) are loved by children, as well as beginner and experienced gardeners. They really are the cheery faces of the garden world. Their clear, bright colours and friendly demeanour are very appealing, and as easy annual plants, they are a delight to grow. They come in just about every hue imaginable and in two size categories, the larger-flowered pansy and the more diminutive viola. Some, but not all, have the distinctive 'face' that helps bees to find the pollen and nectar at the centre of the flower. If you remove the spent flower heads, these fun friends will bloom throughout the growing season (although do let some late flowers form seed; see opposite).

Pansies are among the few plants in temperate gardens that can be in flower just about all year round. Some varieties are bred to send up the occasional flower in the midst of winter, and the more diminutive viola flowers tend to withstand wind, rain and frost better than the pansy's bigger blooms. I plant up tubs at the front door every autumn to provide cheer through the winter, often restricting myself to two complementary colours to maximize the effect. Violas can go almost anywhere, and some have even taken up semi-permanent residence in my rockery; I use others more conventionally to provide a carpet underneath larger shrubs and roses in the height of summer. The larger pansy flowers are prone to damage by slugs, particularly in clay soils, but if you put them in hanging baskets and tubs, they will be protected and you will find it easier to deadhead them regularly to keep the display looking fresh.

Food for thought

'Pansy' comes from *pensée*, the French word for 'thought'. In the language of flowers, to give someone a pansy was to demonstrate that they were constantly in your thoughts. The flower's old name, 'heartsease', also suggests its positive role in affairs of love.

Phyto Filters
Make green screens and hedges as air filters

Vehicle traffic and industrial processes result in pollution and reduce the quality of the air we breathe (see pages 24–5). The only answer to poor air quality is to remove the sources of pollution, namely poor industrial practices and vehicles reliant on fossil fuels, but well-designed plantscapes can mitigate some of the problems in the short term. I say 'well-designed' because the idea is for the plants to block and filter poor-quality air, not inhibit it from dispersing. Both the type and the location of the plants are important. Plants that act as a barrier, such as hedges or shelter belts, are better than those that have a spreading canopy and hem in the pollution (such as an avenue of large trees, the canopies of which create an 'umbrella' effect along an entire road). For anyone living next to a major road, the best response is to cultivate a hedge 3–4m (10–13ft) high along the edge of the property or garden.

The plants that are most beneficial at trapping pollutant particles are those with lots of very fine leaves (and therefore a large total surface area), rough leaves, hairy leaves or waxy leaves. So a tight-knit hedge of evergreens, such as *Cupressus macrocarpa, Viburnum*

Leafy green suburbs: not just pretty

Telomeres are short sections of DNA that protect our chromosomes in the cell nucleus, and they are indicators of stress. The length of these organic 'bits of string' provides clues about our lifestyle and how much exposure our cells have had to inflammation and oxidative stress. They are effectively a cellular record book of stressful events. Research suggests that telomeres become frayed and shorten when humans are exposed to adverse environments, including those with greater air pollution. Shorter telomeres reflect higher susceptibility to disease and a shorter life expectancy. Recent studies have shown direct relationships between telomere length and surroundings. Living in close proximity to green space correlates with longer (and therefore healthier) telomeres.

Plants that act as
a barrier, such as
hedges or shelter
belts, are better
than those that
have a spreading
canopy and hem
in the pollution

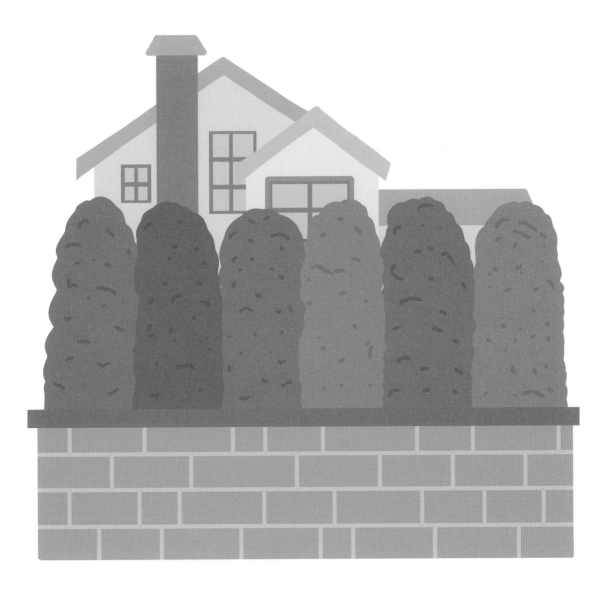

tinus 'Eve Price', *Ilex aquifolium, Elaeagnus × ebbingei, Escallonia laevis* 'Gold Ellen', *Griselinia littoralis, Hedera* and *Taxus baccata*, will screen out some particulates. If there is more space, consider a wider shelter belt composed of species such as pine (*Pinus sylvestris* and *P. pinea*), the hairy-leaved *Sorbus aria* 'Lutescens', *Arbutus unedo, Buddleia davidii, Viburnum lantana* and perhaps one or two cultivars of *V. carlesii*. The last-named have the bonus of blooms with a divine scent.

To provide blockage nearer ground level, add low-growing *Cistus, Euonymus fortunei* (the cultivar 'Emerald 'n' Gold' is particularly striking) and the silver *Brachyglottis* 'Sunshine', with its yellow daisy flowers. If there is enough light left after planting all these shrubs and trees, add the tall stems of *Tithonia rotundifolia*, with its bright burnt-orange blooms, yellow *Verbascum* or *Helianthus*, or multi-hued hollyhocks (*Alcea*); all have very useful rough or hairy leaves. Overall, the objective is to maximize the amount of plant material between you and the source of the pollution.

Research is ongoing as to what types of plant are best at 'scrubbing' different pollutants (that is to say, removing them from the air), and this is important to ensure we create complementary planting that is highly functional in cleaning the air. But such planting should also result in attractive and well-loved landscapes, especially if

Pollen: not to be sneezed at

Plants can improve local air quality, but they can also reduce it. Anyone who suffers from hayfever will know the misery that allergic reactions to plant pollen can cause. Humans are sensitive to both grass and certain types of tree pollen, most usually trees in the Betulaceae (birch) family. Although hayfever can be debilitating in early summer (from tree pollen) or midsummer (grass pollen), for a few individuals it can lead to more serious and potentially life-threatening asthma. The irony is that the allergenicity of *Betula* pollen seems to get worse when combined with poor air quality derived from pollution. Such interaction is complex. Scientists are seeking solutions by identifying which proteins in the pollen people are most allergic to, with the idea in the long term of selecting and planting only those *Betula* genotypes that have low levels of these particular proteins.

Green screens: observing the unforeseen

The developing lungs of children are particularly vulnerable to the effects of poor-quality air, and schools have been instrumental in trying to improve air quality in their environs, for example by encouraging parents to switch off their car engines while waiting to pick up their children. Some have gone further, and one of the Ph.D students in my department worked with a school in Sheffield to develop a planted 'green screen' around the school playground. The screen included functional plants, such as eastern white cedar (*Thuja occidentalis*), ivy (*Hedera helix*) and bamboo (*Phyllostachys nigra*), as well as less functional but attractive lavender (*Lavandula angustifolia*) and *Verbena bonariensis*.

This was known as the BREATHE project, and the primary aim was to give children a degree of protection against pollutants from the surrounding roads. But pupils, teachers and parents also suggested that it had wider, unforeseen benefits, including making the playground more attractive and safe, increasing opportunities for play, promoting mental well-being, bringing parents and teachers together around a 'common cause', allowing children to be better connected to nature, raising environmental awareness (in both pupils and parents), and even increasing enrolment at the school.

we want people to care for it both now and in the future. When recommending plant communities for specific benefits, such as air quality, I always introduce a few less 'functional' plants too, simply to provide greater diversity and a stronger aesthetic appeal. We need more than bland, functional 'bio' cladding or filters; we want these landscapes to be truly multifunctional, dynamic and biologically rich. That's where the greatest benefits lie (see above).

Health Benefit
Attention Restoration

This concept, outlined by the psychologists Rachel and Stephen Kaplan in the late 1980s, indicates that through office work and other aspects of modern life, humans are required to concentrate for prolonged periods – known as 'directed attention'. If this is not relieved, it results in fatigue and then stress. However, the natural world provides an antidote to this directed attention and allows us to unwind. There are four elements that promote this process of relaxation:[13]

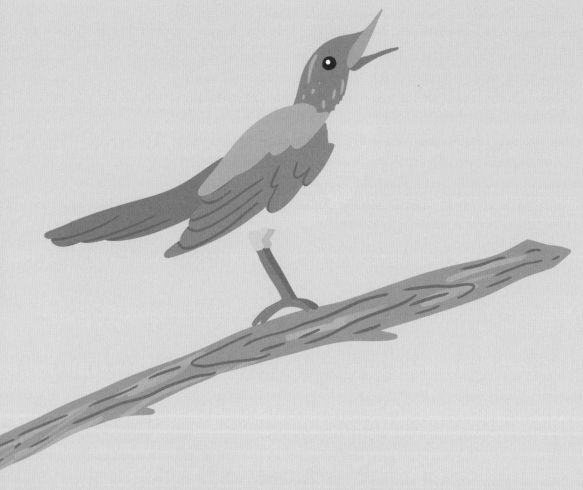

Being away Being physically but also mentally removed from the source of stress. A ten-minute walk in the garden after being on the computer for an hour could be restorative, but so could just switching off the computer and daydreaming about a forthcoming holiday.

Soft fascination Being stimulated by objects that interest the brain but don't overtax it. The natural world is full of these – colourful flowers, leaves blowing in the wind, birdsong, the movement of water in a stream – all of which distract the brain from any problems besetting it.

Extent An environment or activity that allows you to feel totally immersed and engaged. The environment should not provide anything too surprising, and it should make sense to you. Some highly artificial built environments do not make sense because of the amount and complexity of information the brain is receiving. Natural objects and shapes, such as pebbles, leaves and coastal scenes, seem not to overexcite the brain in the same way. Extent is important in allowing soft fascination to occur.

Compatibility A place or activity that allows you to feel joy, and that you are comfortable with. Personal preference can play a part here. Doing an activity that is new or excessively challenging is less restorative than doing one you are familiar and at ease with. For example, cycling down a familiar leafy country lane might be comfortable and relaxing, whereas being asked to drive a tractor for the first time down the same lane might be exhilarating, but not necessarily restorative.

31 | Birds by the Back Door
Use planting to encourage birds into the garden

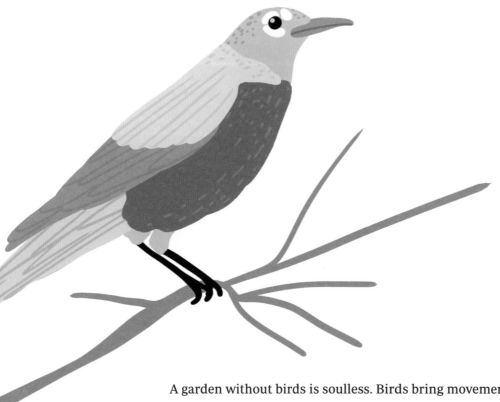

A garden without birds is soulless. Birds bring movement, vitality, drama and often colour, and if you are patient and able to devote a few minutes a day to observing them, you will quickly become hooked on their antics and look forward to their appearances. Once you get your 'eye' in and begin to observe the nuances of their behaviour, you will find their lives fascinating. Never mind kitchen-sink dramas, bird-table dramas are every bit as gripping.

Birds see your garden as real estate and have the same questions as you when considering an ideal home. Is it secure? Warm and cosy in the winter? A good place to raise a family? What are the neighbours like? Are the dining opportunities good? And just as humans might have preferences based on personality and desires, so will

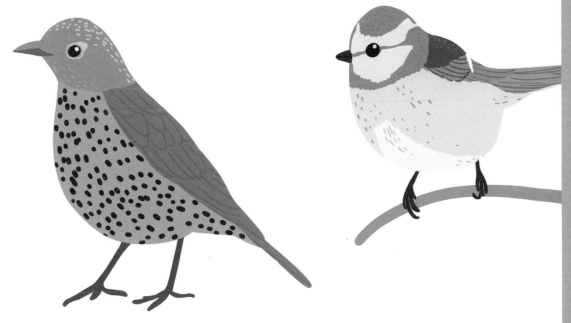

the various bird species. Some sociable types (house sparrows and starlings come to mind) like a communal location, a place to hang out with their mates, while others (robins and blackbirds, including the red-winged types of North America) are more particular about the company they keep, and would rather not have their neighbours too close. Some (wrens and dunnocks) like basement apartments and prefer to skulk around a few metres from ground level, whereas for others (tawny owls and great spotted woodpeckers) only the penthouse suite will do. Northern cardinals have become 'city slickers', preferring town over country; they need woodlands but seem to prefer urban ones, which are a little warmer in winter and provide ready access to backyard feeding stations. In Australia, many parrots (and other bird species) are reliant on large, old trees for nesting cavities. This means that species such as rainbow lorikeets and eastern rosella have aristocratic tastes and demand grand old real estate if they are to do well.

The bird feeder is central to bird life in the garden. Place feeders somewhere you can observe the birds easily, but make sure they are also in a safe spot for the birds themselves. If you observe birds carefully, you will notice that they never stay in one place for too long, and are constantly moving their heads or keeping a lookout for danger. They are 'flighty' by nature, and need to be to survive. Life for a small garden songbird is high-octane, and they must keep moving or they will end up as someone's dinner.

Provide security for your feathered companions with appropriate planting. A dense, well-branched shrub growing 2–3m (6–10ft) from the feeder is superb, and will form the secure 'base camp' for approaching and retreating from the feeder itself. Evergreen shrubs, such as holly (*Ilex aquifolium* or *I. × altaclerensis*) and *Elaeagnus*, provide sanctuary during the winter months, when other shrubs are leafless. Variegated gold or silver cultivars of both genera can be used to brighten a dark corner, such as *E. × ebbingei* 'Limelight'.

Shrubs and small trees are also sources of food for fruit-eating birds. I have planted about 20 types of rowan (*Sorbus*) in my own garden, not just for their attractive bright berries (see chapter 27) and autumn foliage, but also because they act as bird magnets. The resident blackbirds and song thrushes tend to gobble the orange berries of the native rowan, *S. aucuparia*, but are more fussy over the pink-and-white-berried Asiatic rowans. The berries of these species (such as *S. cashmiriana*, *S. pseudohupehensis* 'Pink Pagoda' and *S. vilmorinii*) are therefore retained for longer in winter and act as a lifeline for migratory birds. Keep a sharp lookout, though; flocks of migrants, such as fieldfares and redwings, will descend en masse into your garden, but move on again quickly after taking their fill of the berries. If you are really lucky, you may be treated to a flock of spectacular beige and orange waxwings, another example of exclusivity enhancing the wow factor. Don't limit yourself to rowans; other berry-bearing plants vital to birds are *Viburnum*, *Cotoneaster*, crab and

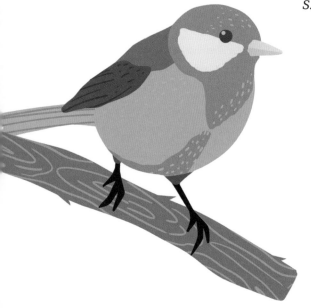

edible apples (*Malus*), *Prunus*, spindle (*Euonymus europaeus*), elder (*Sambucus*), hawthorn (*Crataegus*), ivy (*Hedera*), *Berberis* and *Pyracantha*.

Young birds need to grow fast, and even those species that normally eat grain or fruit will need a source of protein for their young. That means insects and other invertebrates. If you have space, include native plants, which accommodate many insects and their juicy larvae. Leaving a small patch of ground at the end of the garden 'vacant' for native plants can be a blessing in this respect (see chapter 35).

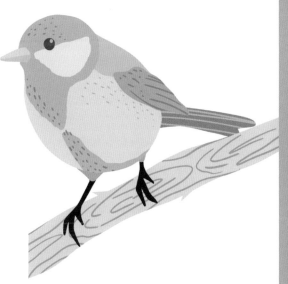

Birds as lifesavers?

Many people find birdwatching fundamental to better mental health, and it has even helped to bring some back from the brink of suicide. The New Economics Foundation cites five mechanisms that improve mental health, and birdwatching (along with other biophilic activities) can help you to achieve these. The points, which are brought home elegantly by Joe Harkness in his thought-provoking book *Bird Therapy* (2019), are:

1 **Taking note** Be aware of your surroundings, notice details and take time to enjoy the present. Watching and appreciating bird life entails these things.

2 **Learning** Improve your understanding, widen your horizons, don't get stuck in 'your bubble', and set goals to acquire new information. Once you have an initial interest in birds, you will want to find out more.

3 **Being active** Engage with physical activity, move around. Search for birds and visit new places in the process.

4 **Connecting** This can mean empathizing with the birds themselves and with their challenges, but also making new friends and acquaintances through your hobby. Join local birding groups or chat to other birders at nature reserves.

5 **Giving** Pass on that knowledge by giving time to someone new to the hobby. Help the birds themselves through feeding them and providing habitat. Giving is great therapy since it is about someone or something else benefiting, rather than dwelling on your own situation and problems. You will get a buzz from helping others, whether human or avian.

32 | **Get the Blood Pumping**
Plant hot-coloured *Rudbeckia*,
Helenium and *Hemerocallis*

Some natural features
excite and enliven us,
and this is known as
positive affect

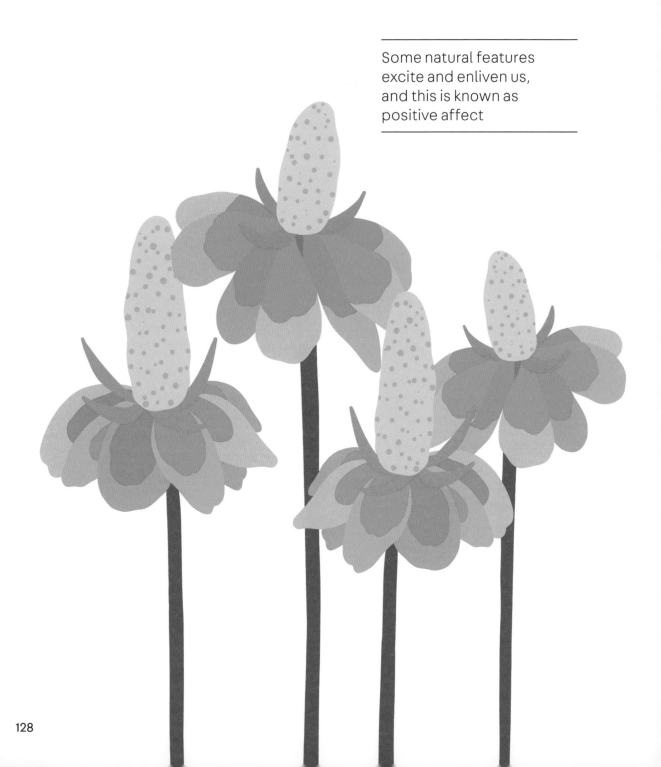

We often associate the natural world with a calming effect, and with providing us with time and space to de-stress. But some natural features do almost the opposite; they excite and enliven us, and this is known as positive affect. These are the jaw-dropping moments that you might associate with seeing a river in torrent, a red sunrise over the desert or a flock of stunning, brightly coloured birds. Such experiences get the pulse racing and leave you with a wonderful memory and a smile on your face. Regularly experienced, such positive events build up mental resilience.

Plants and garden features can promote positive affect, too. Indeed, they can be designed precisely to achieve this – to make you stop, smile and feel good. Strong colours, bold shapes and mass effects are key; there is little room for subtlety. The strong, hot colours are the reds, yellows and oranges, of course. Clear hues provide the brightest impact, but darker or less clear tones can be added to the mix for dramatic effect through contrast. For example, an exuberant yellow can be played off against a deep ruby-red or a sultry, dark chocolate-brown.

Several of the mid- and late summer-flowering herbaceous perennials and annuals have marvellously hot colours. Many are in the aster (daisy) family (such as black-eyed Susan, *Rudbeckia*; tickseed, *Coreopsis*; sneezeweed, *Helenium*; and sunflower, *Helianthus*), and we associate them with North American prairies in high summer. They can be augmented with a wide selection of daylily cultivars (*Hemerocallis*) and *Dahlia* in a bright array of golds, ambers, reds and purples. A number of the true species are vigorous, but some cultivars possess more tempered habits, and will fit into small borders and even pots.

Rudbeckia fulgida var. *sullivantii* 'Goldsturm' is a mainstay for this fiery border community, with its bright-yellow flowers like mini suns transposed from a child's drawing. It will bloom from midsummer until the onset of winter, with a bit of luck. To provide contrast of shape, consider one of the yellow coneflowers or Mexican

Seeing amber: orange as a stimulator

One of my Ph.D students carried out a survey to find out how people respond to colour when viewing flowers in an informal setting such as a meadow or prairie. Almost 700 people responded to the survey, and the most popular flower colours were compositions based on white, blue or orange. Blue was seen as a soothing, relaxing colour (see 18), but orange was popular for its cheering effect and was linked to terms such as 'bright', 'warm', 'uplifting' and 'happy'. Interestingly, white flowers were popular and enlivened the emotions of some people, while relaxing others. Easy-to-grow annual plants with bright mid-orange flowers, such as the California poppy (*Eschscholzia californica*) and pot marigolds (*Calendula officinalis*) can be used to brighten up odd spaces in the garden, and will even self-seed in gravel or between pavers. Whether intentionally planted or not, they are a very welcome sight indeed.

hats (*Ratibida pinnata*), with flowers that do indeed look rather like sombreros. For eye-searing oranges, explore one of the *Helenium* cultivars, such as 'Sahin's Early' or 'Chipperfield Orange', or an *Echinacea*, such as 'Orange Skipper'. Some of the ball and cactus dahlias, such as 'Striped Vulcan', look almost aflame themselves. For red, *Echinacea* (such as 'Sombrero Salsa Red' or even the double 'Double Scoop Cranberry', with its almost ball-like flower) is useful. I have a soft spot for red *Hemerocallis*, though, and 'Chicago Apache', with its fuller flower, and 'Crimson Pirate', with narrower petals, are both great in limited spaces. All fires have their charred embers, of course, and if you want to tone down these vibrant colours, the more muted shades of certain sunflowers (such as the maroons of *Helianthus annuus* 'Moulin Rouge' and 'Claret', or the fawns and browns of 'Earthwalker' and 'Little Becka') are worth bearing in mind.

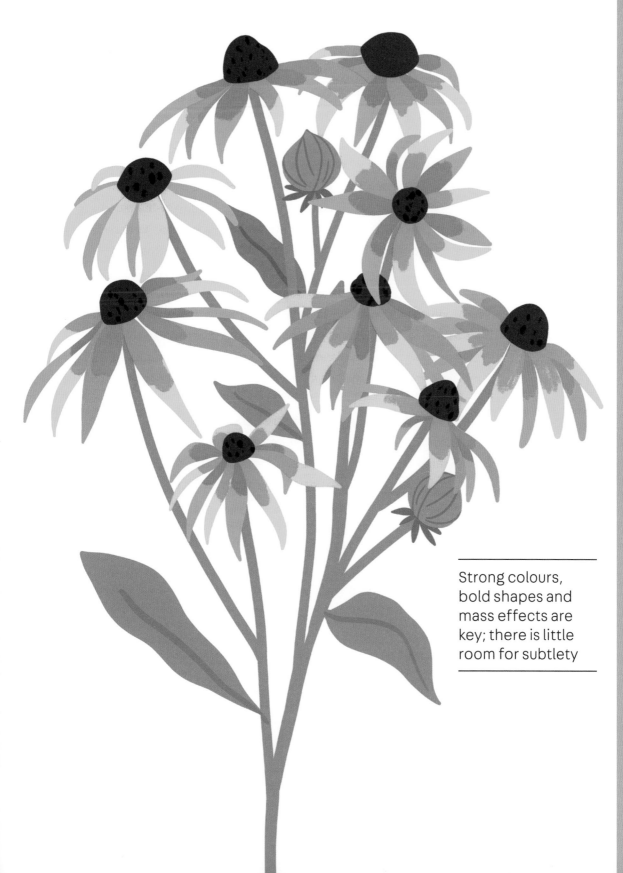

Strong colours,
bold shapes and
mass effects are
key; there is little
room for subtlety

33 | Flags of Flame
Light up the garden with tulips

Snowdrops, crocuses and daffodils usher in spring (see chapter 48), but the real party starts with the tulips (*Tulipa*). These herald the warmth of summer, and their strong primary colours awaken the senses and are a delight to view. Tulip flowers usually present themselves in clear monotones of red, yellow, purple, white and orange, but they also come in striking striped or bicoloured varieties. Indeed, it is the range of colours that makes this genus so popular, and of course the extensive tulip fields of the Netherlands are one of the floral wonders of the world. Whether displayed en masse or as an individual flower, the tulip genuinely lifts the spirits.

Tulip flowers vary in size and shape, from the large Darwin types to the petite alpine species, as single- or double-cup flowers, and with fringed or plain edges. Perhaps the most striking are the varieties with 'breaks' or streaks in the petals, including the Rembrandt and Parrot tulips. Varieties such as 'Flaming Flag' (white with purple stripes), 'Spring Green' (white and green), 'Groenland' (pink and green), 'Carnival de Rio' (red and white), 'Prinses Irene' (orange and purple) and 'Helmar' (red and yellow) are very dramatic. The true parrot or feathered tulips look as if someone has gone along the edges of the petals with crimping shears. Examples to look out for are 'Blue Parrot' (purply blue), 'Estella Rynveld' (red and white), the dramatic 'Black Parrot' and the crumpled mass of petals that is 'Flaming Parrot' (yellow with flickers of red veining).

If you prefer the more classic look, the hourglass-shaped fluted or lily-flowered types may appeal. 'Lasting Love', for example, comes in burgundy – an apt colour for the wineglass shape of the bloom. I grow most of these types in pots and tubs in prominent places, such as at the edge of the lawn, where they can be viewed from the house. Once the flowers are over, the pots can be moved somewhere less conspicuous but still in full light, to allow the foliage to grow on and die down naturally. Tulips must recuperate their energy if they are to flower well the following year, but if you don't have the time or space to encourage this, you can always buy more bulbs the following autumn – they are relatively inexpensive.

Tulips can of course be grown directly in the ground, so are suitable for flower borders, alongside shrubs and as companions for herbaceous flowering plants, as long as their own foliage is not shaded out. They resent heavy, waterlogged soil, so if you garden on clay, grow them in a raised bed. Whatever your soil, make sure you put gravel or free-draining compost in the base of the planting hole before inserting the bulb. By choosing moderately vigorous varieties

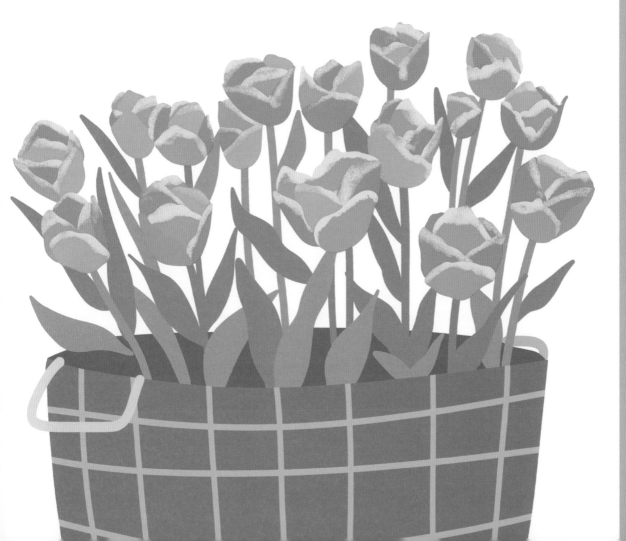

(white 'Hakuun', deepest purple 'Queen of Night', 'Red Revival', 'Pink Impression', 'Yellow Emperor' and 'Apricot Beauty', among many possibilities), you will achieve a recurring display over a number of years, although not every bulb will necessarily flower each year. To give yourself the best possible start, make sure you select the largest bulbs possible in each category. For the larger-flowered types, such as Darwin, Triumph and Single-Early, look for bulbs that are at least 10cm (4in) in circumference at the broadest point. These have more reserves and will have a flower bud. Smaller bulbs, which are often put into mixed multipacks, may take a year or two to produce a flower.

You can buy tulips as early as the end of summer, but if you do so, it is best to store them in a cool place with the bag open or well ventilated, and plant in November (late April or early May in the southern hemisphere). Plant the bulbs so that they are at a depth at least three times the height of the bulb itself. Removing the spent flower heads (but not the leaves) will help to build up reserves in the bulb for next year's flower display.

Some of the most robust and strong-growing varieties, including Darwin types such as 'Apeldoorn' (red), 'Purple Pride' (mauve-purple) and 'Golden Apeldoorn' (yellow), can be planted in meadows or lawns. Although this constitutes an ecological 'battlefield', since grasses are very effective competitors for nutrients and water, the tulips can survive from one year to the next, as long as you allow

Keukenhof: a delight to the eye

Keukenhof, between Amsterdam and The Hague, displays in the region of 800 different tulip varieties each year, representing the planting of a staggering 7 million bulbs each autumn. The garden prides itself on being unique each year in its theme and allied floral displays. All the bulbs are donated by commercial tulip growers, and in effect the garden is a living nursery catalogue. It's not just tulips, either; it is a showcase for many other spring bulbs, too. Keukenhof is said to be the world's largest flower garden, and it's like a sweetshop window for those with a passion for bright and joyous spring flowers.

A lawn full of these beauties is a spectacular sight

the leaves to die down naturally. Growing them in this way is called 'naturalizing', but it does mean leaving the lawn grass to grow long for this period, or at least mowing around the tulips. A lawn full of these beauties is a spectacular sight and, I would argue, worth having an unruly lawn for a bit. Naturalized bright-red tulips always remind me of this species' homeland (Western and Central Asia), where the true species, such as *T. montana* and *T. praestans*, carpet the mountain passes.

In countries such as Iran, Turkmenistan, Uzbekistan and Turkey, the tulip is still loved and revered for its beauty and symbolism. The red symbol at the centre of the Iranian flag is said to mimic the tulip, and legend has it that red tulips flower where religious martyrs have shed their blood. But when talking about tulips, you really can't get away without passing comment on the Netherlands. Horticulture is big business there, and the tulip is near the top of that business. It is estimated that the Netherlands exports about €220 million-worth of cut tulip flowers and bulbs every year. The bulb fields are on Europe's tourist trail, attracting millions of visitors for the 8–10 weeks the main crops are in flower. Tourists wanting to take photographs of friends and families in a colourful field rarely tiptoe through the tulips carefully enough, though, and significant damage can result to the crops. For this reason, the Dutch tourist trade actively promotes the gardens at Keukenhof (see opposite) as a one-stop shop to see most of the tulip varieties at close range, and in more natural and relaxing settings than the production fields can provide.

Health Benefit
Human Microbiome

The philosopher René Descartes famously said, 'I think, therefore I am', a statement that means: if I am thinking, I must also be existing. But did he get it right? Should it not be, 'We think, therefore we are'? Human individuals see themselves as a single identity, but in reality we are effectively a walking commune. Only 43 per cent of 'our' cells are human; the rest are microbial interlopers: bacteria, viruses, fungi and archaea. The non-human-to-human ratio gets worse when we compare genomes; we are outnumbered 1,000 to 1 in terms of genes embedded in our own bodies. Throw in the fact that of our own DNA, only about 5 per cent is 'uniquely human', and one begins to feel feel that our bodies are a bit like an entire walking ecosystem, rather than an autonomous individual personality.

'Personality' is an important term here, since scientists believe that these intrinsic 'little friends' affect the way we think and feel. The greatest concentration of human microbial symbionts dwell in our oxygen-deprived bowels (the gut). But to use the word 'dwell' is to do them a disservice; they work very hard to process our food, reduce our sensitivity to allergens, enhance our immunity and, by regulating hormones, protect our mental health. Moreover, we inoculate our gut microbiome by breathing in or ingesting these beneficial microbial organisms. These 'good' microbiota are closely associated with green and biologically rich environments.[14] Thus, to maximize exposure to the beneficial groups, it seems we need to be in regular contact with diverse plant and soil-organism communities, or our immunity and mental health will suffer.

This concept is linked to the 'hygiene hypothesis', which suggests that after birth a baby's immune response is impaired by being brought up in an extremely clean household of the kind that is now so prevalent in the developed world. Essentially, such an environment is too clean to challenge and educate the baby's natural immune system. The dysfunctional immune system therefore means that the developing child is prone to allergies, such as asthma and food intolerances.

Studies carried out in Finland back up these theories. The addition of forest soil to kindergarten play areas altered the skin and gut microbiomes of the children who attended.[15] Corresponding changes in the children's immunity were observed within a month. These included alterations to plasma cytokines (proteins involved in cell-to-cell signalling and often linked to regulating immunity and inflammation responses), an increase in bacterial diversity (Gammaproteobacteria) and more regulatory T-cells in the blood, suggesting that 'playing in dirt' had stimulated immunoregulatory pathways. (Regulatory T-cells control the immune response to self and foreign particles, and help to prevent autoimmune disease.) But it's not just babies and children who benefit from playing in nature. Being in nature allows adults to top up their health-giving skin and gut microbiomes, too.

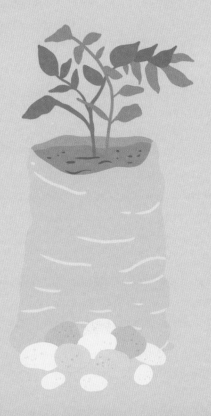

34 Fabulous Fruit
Grow red fruit in unusual places

'Strawberries, cherries and an angel's kiss in spring
My summer wine is really made from all these things.'

The 1960s song 'Summer Wine' by Lee Hazlewood summarizes the seductive qualities of many red summer fruit. These include the raspberry, tayberry, loganberry (all *Rubus*), plum (*Prunus domestica*), red grape (*Vitis vinifera*), redcurrant (*Ribes rubrum*), strawberry (*Fragaria × ananassa*) and sweet cherry (*Prunus avium*), and all have a unique and vibrant taste. The flavour of the fresh fruit straight off the bush is fantastic, and you sometimes have to stop yourself from eating the entire crop there and then, rather than harvesting them for a mealtime, as intended. Of course, the plant is 'hoping' that you will feel this irresistibility; it has spent a lot of energy packaging its seeds into a sweet morsel to entice you (or some other omnivore or frugivore) to ingest it and disperse the seed across the landscape. The attractive red colour is no accident either, and is the signal to say 'this parcel is ripe and ready to go.'

Red fruit provides many health benefits and is full of anthocyanin flavonoids. Anthocyanins are antioxidants and suppress the activity of free radicals in our cells (see chapter 14 and pages 76–7). The phytochemicals and fibre that red fruit provides help to protect us against cancer, improve blood circulation and prevent blood from clotting excessively, as well as supporting a healthy heart. So you can gorge on these supreme red morsels with a clear conscience.

I strongly suggest that you grow some of these delicious fruit if space allows. You do not need a formal fruit area or special cage; just consider a spare sunny location that could do with a flush of greenery. Strawberries such as 'Emily' (early cropping), 'Cambridge

Favourite', 'Redgauntlet' (both mid-season), 'Fenella' and 'Symphony' (both late season) could be allowed to tumble out of a window box. Some new strawberry varieties, such as 'Toscana', have ornamental value, too, with attractive deep-pink flowers interspersed with the fruit. This variety will crop consistently from midsummer through to early autumn. Redcurrants such as 'Jonkheer van Tets' and 'Stanza' can be grown by a drainpipe, or remove a slab or two from the patio and put in a thornless raspberry, such as *Rubus* 'Sweet Sunshine'.

Cherry varieties now come in the dwarf or patio form, removing the need to scale ladders (trees in traditional cherry orchards could be 10–15m/33–50ft high). The height and vigour of fruit trees are determined by the rootstock on to which they are grafted, and

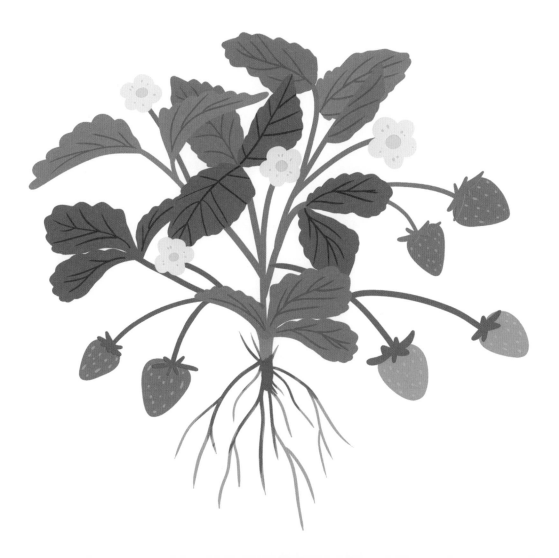

Free radicals: not a new political movement

Our bodies are not perfect and the environment around us is not perfect. Through our body's biochemical processes, we produce 'reactive' oxygen- or nitrogen-based molecules known as free radicals. These exist independently within our tissues, but are reactive in nature owing to the presence of an unpaired electron. Thus they are looking to 'meet' another molecule and either steal one of their electrons or, more generously, donate their electron to the new molecule (acting as an oxidant). Either way, they disrupt the natural order of the other molecule – and that molecule may be a key part of your cell nucleus or one of its protective membranes. Free radicals are non-discriminatory and can interfere equally with DNA, protein, carbohydrate and lipid (fat) structures. Our body can cope with a certain amount of free-radical activity, but if these molecules become too common, they overwhelm the body's defence mechanisms, triggering ailments and disease.

Red fruit provides many
health benefits and is full
of anthocyanin flavonoids

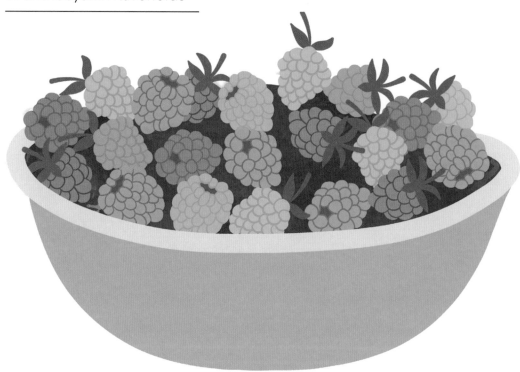

a good semi-dwarfing rootstock for cherry is Gisela 5, so look for varieties grafted on to this. For the top part of the cherry (the scion), consider 'Summer Sun', 'Sunburst' and 'Van' for flavour and a juicy texture. Some scions, such as 'Hartland', have a compact habit themselves, so are good for patio use.

Cherries can also be trained as fan-shaped trees tied in against a wall, taking advantage of a warm microclimate in this situation that often encourages rapid and even ripening of the fruit. Wall-trained cherries can be a magnificent sight. If you can keep the birds off, you can have a whole wall of plump, near-black fruit (such as 'Sasha' or the luxuriant 'Kordia'), scarlet 'hearts' ('Sweetheart', 'Celeste', 'Stella' and 'Meteor Korai') or golden-yellow, sometimes red-flecked fruit ('Vega', 'Stardust Coveu'). Slightly confusingly, the yellow and paler red cherries are sometimes referred to as white, but this refers to the colour of the flesh, not the skin. The grand old masters 'Napoleon' and 'Merton Glory' fall into this category. The wall itself acts as a useful anchor for attaching netting to deter birds during the brief ripening period.

Anthocyanin: the protective dye

Anthocyanins are the pigments that give red and purple fruit their colour. They are deemed good for us because they are a form of compound known as an antioxidant. It is antioxidants that provide our antidote to the deleterious effects of free radicals (see opposite). Antioxidants neutralize the behaviour of free radicals essentially by entering into a pact with them to swap electrons, and thus stopping the vital parts of our cells from being targeted and damaged. In this way they protect the integrity of DNA (thereby preventing the formation of cancer cells) and lipids (ensuring the functionality of important organelles, such as arteries).

The environment is key for this biochemical 'warfare' in our bodies. Poor lifestyle, stress, smoking, inactivity, a high-fat diet, exposure to pollution and so on increase the occurrence and activity of free radicals. Conversely, we can maintain our defences by regularly ingesting antioxidants such as anthocyanins.

Make Room for Nature

35

Cherish the weeds and let the grass grow

Gardens reflect wider interests and values, and consequently often express the personality of the gardener. Broadly, gardeners can be divided along three lines when it comes to characteristics and desires. Some see the garden as an extension of the house. If they are tidy-minded at home, they are tidy-minded in the garden. The lawn edges will be neatly trimmed, the bedding plants arranged in carefully thought-out patterns, and the paths kept spotless. The garden is the 'shop window' of a well-run and well-ordered household, and will reflect a desire for order, neatness and control.

Others interpret the garden as a playground and a place to express artistic and creative interests. Such gardens will have quirky

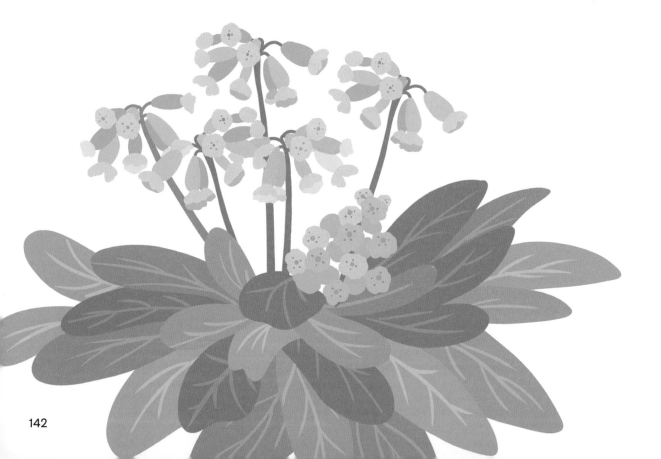

elements. The colours will be chosen to make a bold or reflective statement: a re-creation of a historic garden style, perhaps, or the presentation of a strong central theme. Such design can be inspired by a vast range of topics, and may mirror an interest in the sea, Japanese philosophy or old Victorian hardware. The garden is used in the manner of a canvas, to reproduce ideas. People with a creative nature like this will find their garden immensely stimulating.

The third group see the garden as offering the first steps into the wider natural world. Here starts the extended journey to the Serengeti, the Amazon or the Arctic; all nature is connected, and the garden is the first place where people experience it on leaving home. It is a place to design and be creative in, but it also belongs to others, the snails, the woodlice, the yellow-necked fieldmouse and all their allies. For people with an ecocentric view of the world, this is the chance to have 'Eden on the doorstep'.

It is this last group that will get the most out of allowing nature to 'do its own thing'. Theirs is a relaxed – some might even say untidy – style of gardening. If you feel you are in this ecocentric group, try using the 'guiding hand' rather than the 'controlling hand'. Gardening in this way is about observing nature, making room for other species and noticing the small things – which are often also the best – simply appear. It is a truly biophilic philosophy.

There is no better way to experience biophilia than by reducing the frequency of mowing a lawn, preferably one that has been neglected and has relatively low levels of nutrients in the soil (see chapter 25). In northwestern Europe you will be surprised at how quickly flowers, such as lesser celandine (*Ficaria verna*), creeping buttercup (*Ranunculus repens*) and meadow buttercup (*R. acris*), dandelions (*Taraxacum*), violets (*Viola odorata*) and tormentil (*Potentilla erecta*), appear. Leave the grass for longer between mowing sessions and a short-stature meadow will form, with yellow archangel (*Lamium galeobdolon*), white dead nettle (*L. album*), red dead nettle (*L. purpureum*), betony (*Betonica officinalis*), cowslip (*Primula veris*), field scabious (*Knautia arvensis*), ragged robin (*Lychnis flos-cuculi*) and meadow cranesbill (*Geranium pratense*). The common lawn grasses (*Festuca* and *Agrostis*) will also flower, looking magical when the early dew catches their seed heads.

Note that I said 'guiding hand', however. Stop intervening completely and your lawn may actually lose biodiversity. For example, if the soil is rich in nutrients, you may end up with a patch of nettles (*Urtica dioica*), dock (*Rumex*), bramble (*Rubus fruticosus*) and thistle (*Cirsium arvense*); that's great for invertebrates and small mammals, but these vigorous plants tend to crowd others out, so you will lose a number of the flowering plants. In general terms, plant diversity is optimized by small, infrequent stress events such as drought, lack of key nutrients, or fire, which stop a limited number of very competitive species from dominating the show.

A relaxed style of gardening also allows beautiful 'weeds' to self-seed along pathways and in walls. You may find that red valerian (*Centranthus ruber*), honesty (*Lunaria annua*) and Welsh poppy (*Papaver cambricum*) turn up spontaneously. I carried out an experiment on pansies and violas one year in front of my garage, and ever since, tiny specimens of 'wild-like' *Viola* progeny have appeared between the cracks in the pavers. An unusual appearance of a plant, especially in an unexpected place, can give quite a thrill.

Where possible, encourage the wild flowers that are native to your area. Not only are they usually easier to establish, but also they will be well fitted for the local animals, including pollinators. (In large countries with a range of climates and habitats, look for seeds that suit your specific area. For example, in the United States, seed firms will provide separate collections for the Pacific North-West, Mid-West and Eastern States.) Classics include kangaroo paws (*Anigozanthos*) and *Brachyscome* in Australia, Texan bluebonnet (*Lupinus texensis*) and tickseed (*Coreopsis tinctoria*) in North America, *Anemone coronaria* and *Geranium* in Greece and *Dimorphotheca* and *Gazania* in South Africa.

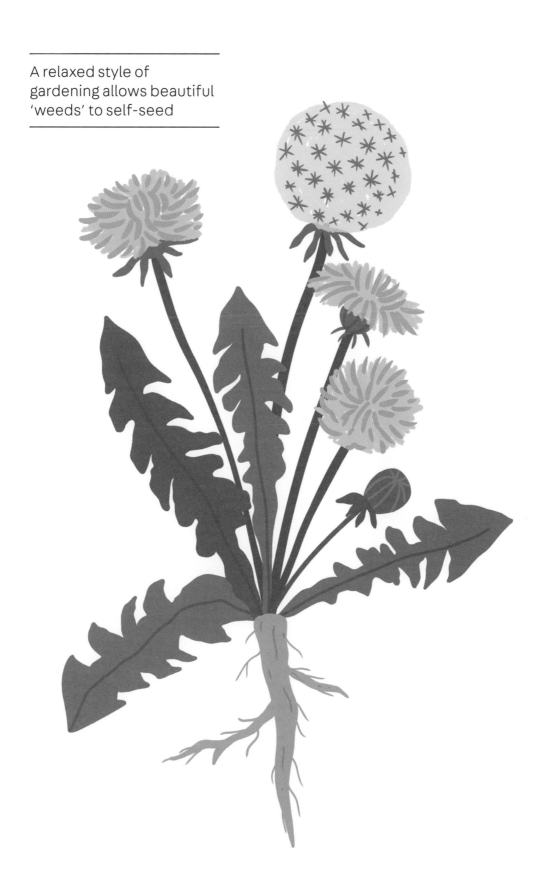

A relaxed style of gardening allows beautiful 'weeds' to self-seed

Close and Personal

36

Create an intimate space around a bench

People who suffer bereavement or trauma often look for intimate, enclosed spaces

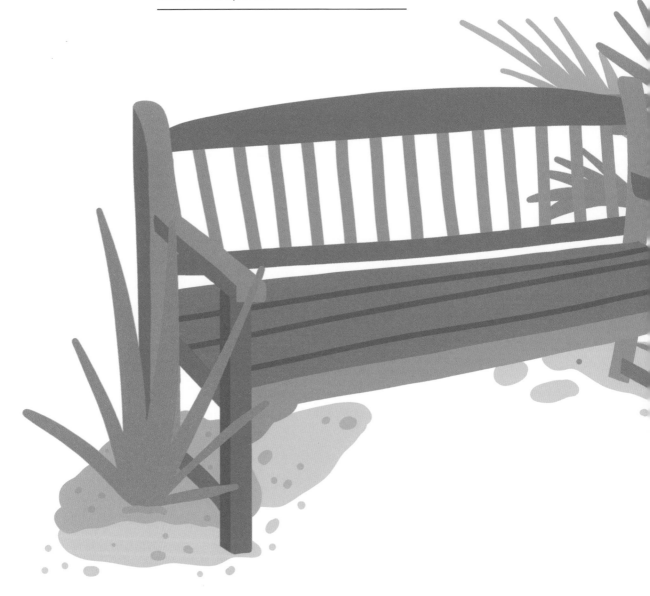

The biophilia theory suggests that humans relate to landscapes that were important in our evolution. An example is the typical urban park, with its open spaces dotted with groups of large trees. Such a landscape is not dissimilar to the savannahs of eastern and southern Africa, where it is thought *Homo erectus* (our first upright ancestor) came out of the forest and started to stroll around. She became upright to see over the tall grass, in the way that baboons sometimes do today to check for danger.

These early hominids were vulnerable to large predators such as lions (and their sabre-toothed 'big cat' equivalents), and were most comfortable when they had shelter and vantage points. Although humans aren't often chased by lions in suburbia nowadays, these are still feelings and landscapes that we can relate to. We like to site seats and other resting places in locations where we feel enclosed and secure, or where we have some view or vantage point. Sometimes in a garden we combine both: the back of the bench 'cuddles up' to the house or garden wall, while the front looks out over the lawn or pond, or perhaps provides a view down a shallow slope. We want to see forwards over the landscape, while ensuring that our backs are protected.

For intimacy, we might want our bench to be enclosed about half to two thirds by physical structure. We desire a concave 'room' shape, and the outer circle might be a low wall, hedging, or an array of pots and containers of flowing, tranquil plants. Medium-sized shrubs are useful in this respect, since they provide intimacy without being overbearing. A concave design might be composed of *Daphne, Ceanothus, Cistus*, Mexican orange blossom (*Choisya ternata*), winter-flowering honeysuckle (*Lonicera fragrantissima*) and lavender (*Lavandula angustifolia*), with subtle, pastel-coloured flowers and soothing perfumes. To add movement, we might incorporate tall Chinese fountain grass (*Pennisetum alopecuroides*) or silver grass (*Miscanthus sinensis* 'Morning Light'), with smaller ornamental grasses such as blue fescue (*Festuca glauca*) and pony-tail grass (*Stipa tenuissima*). If space allows, try a taller evergreen plant with stronger form, such as a conifer, set back from the bench. Serbian spruce (*Picea omorika*), in a slower-growing variety such as 'Peve Tijn', or Colorado blue spruce (*Picea pungens* 'Hoopsii') would be ideal. The key is to make this place as comfortable as possible – a bolthole in times of stress, and a place to wind down when we need peace and quiet.

To complete the biophilic theme, give careful consideration to the landscape and plants that compose the vista from your seated sanctuary. Research has suggested that in North America, children under the age of 12 prefer savannahs over more familiar types of biome, such as coniferous or deciduous forests,[16] so perhaps the view from your secluded bench should include a mix of grasses and flowering perennials with a 'flat-topped' tree in the background. For the latter, you might use a Japanese maple (*Acer palmatum*), with its naturally horizontal structure, or train a Scots pine (*Pinus sylvestris*) to mimic the classic umbrella-shaped thorn trees (*Vachellia tortilis* subsp. *heteracantha*) of the African savannah. Scots pines naturally form a flat 'head' with age, but you can speed this up by judiciously pruning out the leading shoots each spring. This is a common technique in Japan, where gardeners have perfected the art of

Enclosure as sanctuary

People who suffer bereavement or trauma often look for intimate, enclosed spaces. They desire time for themselves and for reflection. If they want company, it may be from only a close family member or trusted friend. Peace, serenity, privacy, familiar surroundings, and features and natural sounds, such as wind or birdsong, are desirable; intrusions, external influences and wider social engagements are usually not welcomed.

'I don't like spiders and snakes': nature or nurture?

The biophilia theory is a controversial one, since it essentially states that we are hardwired to like certain features of the natural world. This does not sit comfortably with the idea of free choice. Ironically, probably the best evidence for biophilia is actually its negative counterpart, biophobia. Many people have a fear of spiders and snakes. This seems logical when we consider that some of these creatures can harm us, but is such behaviour learned or innate?

A study of six-month-old babies in 2017 suggested that it is innate.[17] The babies' pupils dilated when they were presented with images of snakes or spiders, and they did not have the same reaction when viewing fish or flowers. During the experiment, the babies sat on their mother's laps, but the mothers wore dark glasses and could not see the images, so they did not react to them. The infants' dilated pupils were considered a stress reaction, since dilation is associated with the brain's noradrenergic system and is linked to arousal and vigilance.

This suggests that the babies were responding negatively to the spiders and snakes without any influence from their environment, and thus that the response must have been instinctive rather than learned. Others argue, however, that even by the age of six months, babies may have learned from their parents how to react to snakes and spiders. The debate continues.

cultivating young pines so that they appear to be hundreds of years old. Similarly, other trees, including the cedars (*Cedrus*), horizontal junipers (such as *Juniperus squamata*), dogwoods (such as *Cornus controversa*), apples (*Malus*) and cherry plums (*Prunus cerasifera*), can be trained into a convincing flat canopy. This notion of an ancestral or genetic link to savannah landscapes has been reinforced by other studies indicating that people prefer trees with spreading crowns over those with rounded or conical canopies.

37 | Compare and Contrast
Start collecting and comparing plants

Good garden design often depends on a minimalist approach, in which relatively few forms and colours come together to create a unifying, consistent theme. We see such designs in glossy gardening magazines. They are dreamy, wonderful outdoor spaces, so tranquil and elegant. But I do struggle with this concept, at least in practice. I am simply not disciplined enough for such designs. There are too many exciting plants that I want to grow, and any design would not stay minimalist for long under my direction.

People from very different walks of life and cultural backgrounds can find common ground in plants

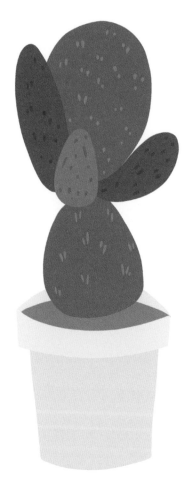
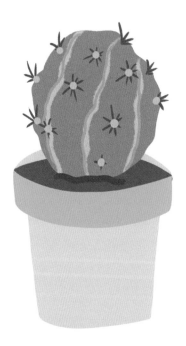

This has something to do with the way I view the world. As a lecturer in training, I learned about student learning styles, about how people accumulate knowledge differently based on their character and how their brain interprets the world around them. I personally depend on a logical-linguistic style of learning. Logical learners like to classify and group information. They make lists of things: car number plates, railway locomotive numbers or, for some of us, plants.

There is great joy to be had from collecting and comparing plants, as we can see if we examine some of the great landscape gardens of the world. Exbury Gardens in Hampshire, southern England, does not have just one or two rhododendrons; it has hundreds of varieties. The Morton Arboretum in Illinois aspires to present every woody plant

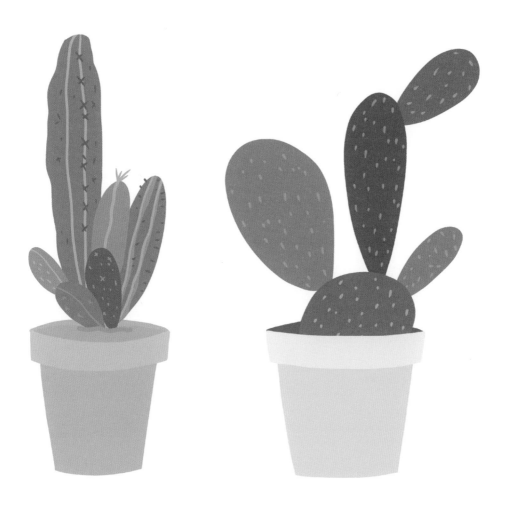

that grows in North America. There is a fascination in collecting and comparing specimens. Some people will spend their life collecting and possessing orchids (sometimes to the detriment of the species in the wild; see chapter 8). But it could equally be *Salvia, Dahlia*, cacti or auriculas. In my case, it tends to be the mountain ashes, *Sorbus*. At a plant nursery, I will make a beeline for the *Sorbus* specimens, ignoring every other tree on display. Only once I have satisfied myself that there is no new *Sorbus* available will I turn my attention to the rest of the nursery's collection. The fact that I have absolutely no more space in my garden for another does not seem to matter. (That is where the logistic approach does not seem to involve much logic.) But this raises an important point. In moderation, the habit can be positive, distracting and therapeutic, but it must not become an obsession.

If you have a similar mindset, find out what you might be interested in. A trip to a local public or botanic garden is a great way to do this, but do start small. The more diminutive flowering plants – among them *Diascia*, pansy (*Viola*), *Dianthus* and *Primula* – are a source of wonder, and usually at pocket-money prices, too. Get into gardening clubs and swap plants with neighbours and those with a similar interest. Plants are great conversation-starters, and you may even gain a wider circle of friends as a result.

If you 'get into' collecting specific types of ornamental plant, you will be joining a movement that goes back a long way. In the Middle Ages

Over the garden fence

Plants are generally seen as a neutral subject of conversation – a bit like the weather. You can make a comment about a flower or garden and not cause offence; indeed, quite the opposite. Most gardeners will be delighted if you compliment their plot. People who would normally ignore each other in the street will stop and pass the time of day if one of them is tidying up the front garden or pruning the roses. The social value of plants and gardening has not been much studied, but the data we have suggest that these topics can be great 'levellers', in that people from very different walks of life and cultural backgrounds can find common ground in plants. It is said that in times gone by the only servant the lord and lady of the manor would treat as an equal was their head gardener, because they genuinely valued his or her knowledge.

Keep an eye out for that rarity

Collectors often desire 'one of each' (colour, for example), the very latest release, a particularly exclusive plant, or a plant that has a special connection for them, perhaps a cultivar their parents grew. The muslin weavers of the town of Paisley in Scotland were world leaders in developing new and colourful strains of pink (*Dianthus*). They developed so-called plain pinks and laced pinks (the latter having fringed petals). One of the few varieties still in cultivation is *D.* 'Dad's Favourite', which has a broad ruby-red line running through the otherwise white petals. I have only a few garden pinks (the obsession has not taken hold on this family yet), but for me, as someone bred and brought up in Paisley, that particular one is a must-have.

in Europe, adherents of certain religions grew plants for symbolic reasons as well as their more practical medicinal properties. The period of tulip mania during the 1630s in the Netherlands is associated with the extravagant breeding and buying of new tulips; many people saw bulbs as an investment, but fortunes were lost when the 'bubble' burst. Country gentlemen and tradespeople joined by a common interest in ornamental plants formed Florists' Societies from the eighteenth century onwards and held annual flower shows or 'feasts'. Societies formed around plants such as carnations and pinks (*Dianthus*), *Chrysanthemum*, auriculas (*Primula*), *Ranunculus* and hollyhock (*Alcea rosea*), not forgetting the tulip (*Tulipa*).

During the Victorian era, working-class people saw plant-collecting as a means of brief respite from the everyday drudgery of industrial life. Miners, steelworkers, weavers and others all had their gardening clubs, many of which were confined to a particular species, and they competed to breed and collect novel colours and shapes. Plant families and their cultivated forms have come and gone as horticultural trends have changed over the years, but the fascination and fashion for collecting itself remains strong.

38 | Taters in a Bag
Grow potatoes in a bag or container

Surely growing your own crops and eating them is the very essence of satisfaction. The sense of achievement is wonderful. This might not always be the most economical or efficient way to feed yourself, but it is immensely enjoyable. Produce straight from the ground or off the bush has the genuinely fresh aroma and taste that often seem to get lost during the commercial harvesting, washing, storage, packing and transportation of crops.

If you have never grown a food crop before, there is nowhere better to start than with the common potato (*Solanum tuberosum*). If garden space is tight, you can grow potatoes successfully in potato grow bags, large tubs or half-barrels. Potato crops are rarely ever started from seed, because it takes too long for the plant to build up enough biomass to produce effective potatoes. Instead we use 'seed potatoes', tubers raised specifically to be free of virus and easily distributed to farmers and gardeners.

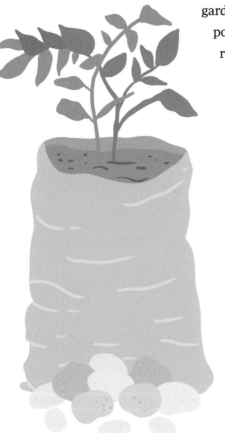

It is a good idea to 'chit' (sprout) these seed potatoes in late winter by placing them in an empty egg box on a windowsill. This encourages the 'eyes' (dormant shoot buds) into active growth. In mid-spring plant the sprouted tubers in containers, trying to avoid knocking off the developing shoots as you do so. The container should be about 50cm (20in) wide and double that in depth. Fill the container half-full with a good-quality growing medium, place three or four tubers on top of this, then add more growing medium to a depth of about 15cm (6in) on top. As soon as new shoots emerge from the substrate, bury them with a further

The sense of achievement is wonderful

15cm of growing medium, and continue in this way until the container is full. This encourages the formation of new tubers from the buried stems. Allow the leaves to grow unhindered through early summer, and your first taters should be ready by midsummer. Small, early potatoes are often used in summer salads; other varieties crop later with larger tubers, which are great for baking.

Potatoes are full of carbohydrates, and are thus one of the staple food crops of the world. They also provide us with vitamins, fibre and minerals such as manganese, and are rich in antioxidant flavonoids, carotenoids and phenolic acids. As with other vegetables (see chapter 14), coloured varieties, such as purple potatoes, can have three or four times more antioxidants than white. Potatoes contain a special type of starch, too. This is known as resistant starch, and tends not to be broken down and absorbed by the body immediately, but rather heads off to the large intestine, where it becomes a source of nutrients for the beneficial microbiota living in the gut (see pages 136–7). Research has linked resistant starch to health benefits, including the reduction of insulin resistance, which in turn improves blood sugar control. It is thought that the resistant starch content of boiled potatoes is enhanced if you store them in the fridge overnight and consume them cold.

The nutritional content of potatoes depends on the variety and the cooking method, but in general, bear in mind that a lot of the nutrients are in the skin. Frying potatoes adds more calories and fat than baking them; as a great fan of French fries, I regret to say it, but boiled and baked potatoes are the healthier option.

Health Benefit
Biophilia

There are evolutionary or even genetic reasons for our love of certain aspects of the natural world (biophilia), or the opposite (biophobia; see page 149). Based on our evolution in the African savannah, we have a preference for certain types of landscape, plant and animal. Studies suggest that we prefer open, sparsely wooded landscapes, green areas with open or running water, and vantage points from where we can scan our surroundings while feeling secure. All this is related to our survival as early hominids.

The origin of the term 'biophilia' is linked to the German psychologist Erich Fromm (1900–1980), but it was popularized by the biologist Edward O. Wilson (1929–2021) through his book *Biophilia* (1984). Wilson argues that our attraction to nature is genetically predetermined and the result of evolution. There are sound reasons why we are drawn to certain natural objects; for example, flowers foretell where fruit will appear (an important point if you are constantly foraging for food across an unpredictable landscape). From an evolutionary perspective, too, early humans who were well connected to landscapes could find water and understood animal life better, and were therefore more

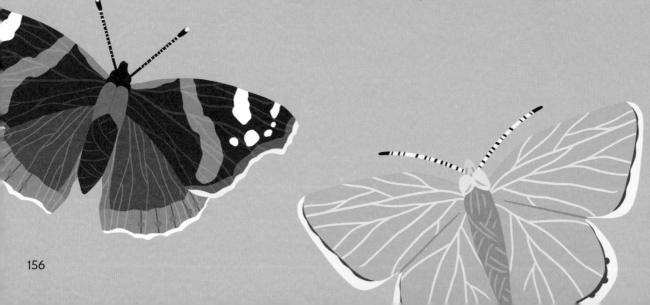

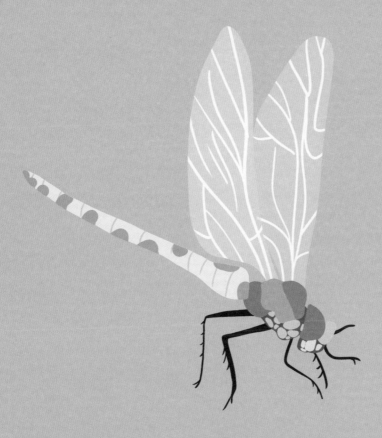

likely to survive and pass on their genes. Even today there is some evidence for this. Children will often make a beeline for the pond or stream when first entering a garden, for example, perhaps even bypassing the gift shop with its allure of ice cream. Water has always been a vital resource, and its legacy in the landscape today is still to draw us in by the way it reflects the light and provides movement. Once at the side of the pond, the first few moments are spent looking for fish or tadpoles, or observing the ducks. These were locations not just to quench our thirst, but also to hunt. Compared to more open bush country, this was the place to find 'easy pickings' or create an ambush (since other animals have to come to drink, too).

The fact that some of these attractions seem intrinsic to us has fostered the notion of a relationship with nature being hardwired into our genes. Our inherent love of gardens and of soft, non-threatening pets may be biophilic relationships.

39 | A View from Above
Climb a tree

There follows a public health warning on tree-climbing. You need a hard hat, a climbing harness, a high-vis jacket, a head for heights and probably a degree in arboriculture – but only if you climb more than 2–3m (6–10ft) high. So I don't advocate that. Indeed, if I were to encourage high tree-climbing without proper training and equipment, I would have to rename this book *50 Ways Plants Could Kill You*!

So please stick to low branches, or small (but sturdy) trees. Tree-climbing is fun, though. Grappling with branches, perching on a bough and sitting quietly while birds come to you, or just enjoying a peaceful moment are all good for your well-being. Children and tree-climbing go hand in hand, or at least they used to; recent surveys suggest that large numbers of us have never climbed a tree. Even if the urge took you today, park laws discourage it in many public spaces, largely through fear of litigation. So another 'rite of passage' disappears off the childhood list.

Seeing the wood in the trees

We are primates, so our brain may still be 'programmed' to deal with arboreal environments; our forward binocular vision, for example, helps us to assess distance when moving through branches and undergrowth. Some studies suggest that physical activity, such as tree-climbing, may prime the brain for further workloads and keep it focused. Experiments have shown that adults who were primed with activities such as navigating forest settings or balancing on a beam had better short-term memory recall than those who did more passive exercise, such as yoga.

This is a pity. Tree-climbing reflects life in that there is risk involved, but also pleasure and a strong sense of achievement. It's an activity that allows children the opportunity to assess risk for themselves. It allows them to test themselves and feel genuine achievement when they reach their limit, and, as importantly, to recognize and respect their limitations when they don't. Tree-climbing and similar calculated risk-taking activities are linked with greater

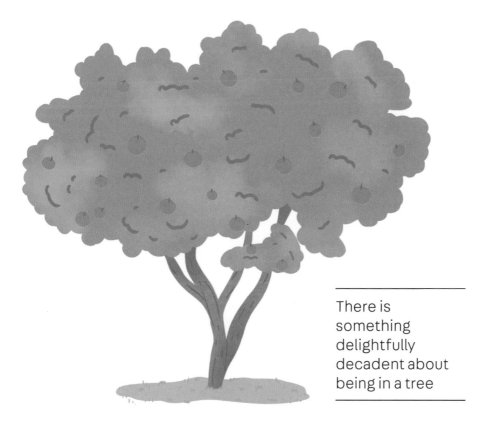

There is something delightfully decadent about being in a tree

physical ability, agility, less sedentary behaviour, longer periods of play, and greater creativity and resilience. Social skills improve when activities are undertaken as a group, and this 'risky play' is linked with better decision-making.

If you haven't climbed a tree for a while (or if you never have), now is the time to give it a shot. There is something delightfully decadent about being in a tree and viewing the passing world while others can't see you. My daughter loved climbing trees because the garden birds did not seem to consider her a threat when she was enveloped in the canopy of a tree, and would venture quite close for her to look at. Alternatively, if you feel the arboreal life is for you, you might want to invest in a hammock. Rocking on a breezy day with the sound of fluttering leaves in your ears is a great form of escapism. Those who have more cash, or excellent carpentry skills, could even consider building a tree house.

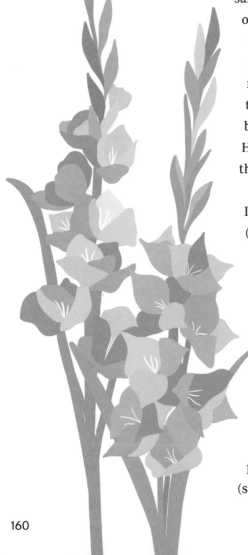

40 Lovable Lilies and Glad Glads
Expand your horizons with exotic blooms

Plants open doors to new worlds. They play on the idea of *extent* – being able to get away from the normal and the familiar – and in effect allow us to escape sources of anxiety or stress. Viewing a simple flower unleashes images of exotic landscapes and exciting adventures, but also links to culture, ways of life and even unfamiliar philosophies. It is a bit like those word-association games that psychiatrists impose on their patients. Think of saffron, for example. What comes to mind? Perhaps one or more of the following: the red stigmas of a beautiful pale pink/purple crocus (*Crocus sativus*), alpine meadows in Greece and the Near East, the most expensive spice in the world (more expensive than gold), the yellow of paella, Cornish saffron buns, tasty curries, a renunciation of material life (in Hinduism and Buddhism), and one of the colours in the Indian national flag.

I see most garden plants in this light. I associate lilies (*Lilium*) with mountainsides in Asia (even though several lily species come from North America or Europe). I imagine my lilies growing at the edge of woodland on a steep slope in China, with a grand frothing, pale-turquoise river in the distance pulsing towards the South China Sea many miles away. Some species fit this scene accurately – *L. taliense* and *L. henryi*, for example – but my imagination is not a purist, and I also see many garden hybrids with not very Chinese names, such as 'Casa Blanca' (pure white), 'Star Gazer' (shocking pink), 'African Queen' (mid-orange) and 'Redhill' (scarlet), in my escapist world.

Lilies like a rich, free-draining soil, and I grow mine in the company of shrubs such as *Rhododendron*, *Camellia* and *Magnolia* to keep the Chinese mountain theme going. They also grow very well in pots, where their requirements can be readily met. A novice to lilies might start with the so-called Asiatic hybrids, which are quite short, with open, upright flowers in a wide range of colours. With time and experience, move on to those with different flower shapes, including the really large-bloomed *L. regale*, 'tiger' lilies such as *L. henryi* (orange), *L. auratum* var. *platyphyllum* (yellow) and the Turk's cap (*L. martagon*).

If lilies transport us to the foothills of the Himalayas, *Gladiolus* species and cultivars take us to the Drakensberg Mountains of South Africa. To be absolutely accurate, today's garden hybrids tend to be larger and more 'in your face' than the naturally occurring species gladioli, but the distinctive sword-shaped leaves and characteristic flower shapes are such an icon of the grasslands of South Africa that you can get away with this association. For that genuine feel of an African grassland, interplant gladioli with a range of attractive ornamental grasses. In such a setting, cultivars such as *Gladiolus* 'Fiorentina' (white with a pink centre), 'Verax' (white with a blue/purple centre), 'Evergreen' (light green), 'Sapporo' (peachy rose with a pale-green throat and red centre) and 'Lumiere' (purple and pink) would provide a subtle, natural feel. To top things off, add other South African icons, such as *Pelargonium* and *Kniphofia*.

Viewing
a simple
flower
unleashes
images
of exotic
landscapes
and exciting
adventures

41 | **Notes of Nature**
Listen to nature in the garden

Natural sounds, in combination with other elements of the natural world, have been linked to decreased stress, annoyance and pain, greater positive affect, and enhanced mood and cognitive performance. They also facilitate the concept of being at one with nature (compatibility) and fully appreciating nature (biophilia). Getting a useful dose of natural soundscapes, then, would seem to be just as important as visualizing the green domain.

Nature makes its voice heard most effectively early in the morning and late in the evening. If you are one of those people whom sleep eludes between 4 and 5am, get up, put the kettle on, grab a coffee and head out into the garden. Assuming you live in a relatively quiet area, you should be in luck. When the rest of the world is quiet, nature makes its presence felt through sound.

The dawn chorus is famous, of course. It peaks in spring, and despite the pressure on some bird species, our little feathered friends can still create a cacophony as the sun makes its appearance. What you hear will depend on where you live, how many trees are close by and whether there are any dense shrubs in your garden (see chapter 31). There is also a sequence, so – as with any music festival – make sure you are there at the right time for your favourite songster. In northern Europe the concert kicks off with skylarks, song thrushes, blackbirds and robins; warblers and wrens tend to breakfast before putting in an appearance and singing their hearts out.

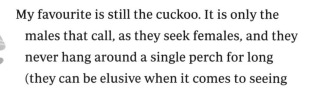

My favourite is still the cuckoo. It is only the males that call, as they seek females, and they never hang around a single perch for long (they can be elusive when it comes to seeing them). The song is as the bird's name sounds ('cuckoo' in English, but also *le coucou* in French). About three males regularly fly around my garden in spring, but one has a distinctly croaky call; he splutters 'cook – ooh, cook – ooh, sqcheee'. Whether that charms the ladies, I don't know.

Every part of the world has its own iconic birdsongs. The eastern whipbird of Australia has, as its name suggests, a song that is similar to the cracking of a whip, and the purple-crested turaco of eastern Africa is reminiscent of a misfiring car. The North American woodpeckers are set apart by their vocalizations, an array of metallic yeep-yeeps and youp-youp-youps, as well as the iconic 'drumming' as they chisel out grubs from dead wood. In places where properties align with remnants of native woodland, such evocative sounds are not uncommon in garden settings.

Birds do not have the monopoly on soothing or intriguing sounds. Some plants love to rustle up a little tune as the wind flows through them (see chapter 47). One of the most famous is the trembling aspen (*Populus tremula*), but other whispering flutterers include the maples (*Acer*) and willows (*Salix*). Running water, with its associated gurgles, is a must for any therapeutic garden. And although I have mentioned the birds, mammals too have their repertoire. Sharp squeaks from the uncut lawn indicate the presence of tiny bank voles, cute rodents with short, blunt noses. Finally, there is the blood-curdling 'call' of a female fox (vixen) in midwinter: an eerie, otherworldly sound, certainly not soothing, but haunting and full of spirit.

42 | **Waking the Senses**
Play with foliage colour

While we often become animated about flowers in the garden matrix, we should consider leaf and stem colour just as much, not least because those features tend to have greater permanence in the landscape. Interestingly, we choose houseplants more in relation to foliage form and structure than to their flowering capabilities, although there are notable exceptions, such as the orchids (see chapter 8).

A relatively uniform foliage colour allows the eye to settle on other traits, such as size, rigidity, texture and form, so green leaves alone can create a dramatic effect. Texture too is important; large, solid, 'bold' leaf shapes are described as coarse-textured, and these seem to stand out and 'come towards' the viewer. By contrast, fine-textured plants, specifically those with small or soft leaves, seem to recede into the landscape. You can make a small space seem larger by grouping coarse-textured plants near the centre and finer ones towards the rear boundary. Texture is also a useful concept when creating contrast between plants. An attractive and stimulating composition of foliage plants might include the bold, star-shaped leaves of *Fatsia japonica* blended with fine foliage from *Carex oshimensis* 'Eversheen', shuttlecock ferns (*Matteuccia struthiopteris*) and *Astilbe chinensis* 'Vision in Pink'.

Strong contrasts of foliage colour can be dramatic. For example, *Cornus alba* 'Aurea' with its golden sprays can be placed against the near black of *Physocarpus opulifolius* 'Diabolo'. Add to this mix the amber flowers of *Crocosmia × crocosmiiflora* 'George Davison' for good late summer effect. At a larger scale, *Cercis canadensis* 'Forest Pansy' (deep red-purple) clashes superbly with the heart-shaped lime-yellow leaves of *Catalpa bignonioides* 'Aurea'. The latter can

We should consider leaf and stem colour just as much, not least because those features tend to have greater permanence

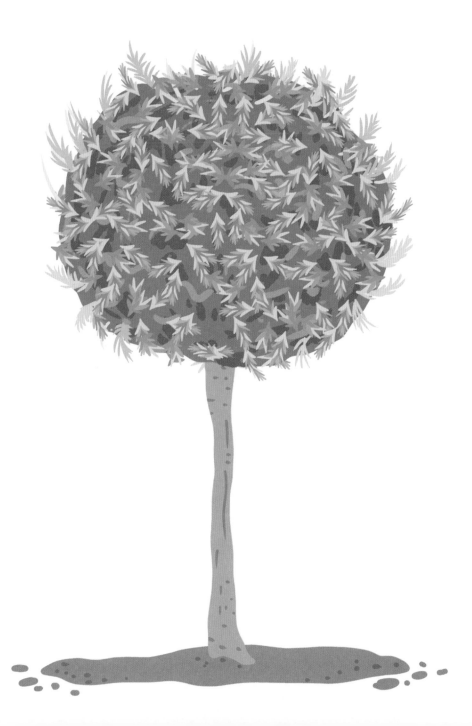

grow large, but it is easily pollarded or coppiced if it gets out of hand. Such strong contrasts and very unsubtle effects bring a smile to my face whenever I encounter them.

Gardeners with less space can have a lot of fun using the numerous brightly coloured forms of coral bells (*Heuchera*). Many new cultivars have been released over the last few years, and there is now a whole palette of deep purples, purple-reds, pink with silver trim, caramels, tawnies, butterscotch and the most vivid lime-green. These are ground-cover plants, so enjoy creating your own floor mosaic.

Preference for plants with variegated foliage comes down to taste. I personally like variegated leaves when the patterns are bold and not too fussy, especially in the green-and-gold combinations. Particularly effective examples, in my view, include *Elaeagnus × ebbingei* 'Gilt Edge', with strictly demarcated green and gold; *Hosta* 'Liberty', with a pale-yellow rim to the leaf that complements rather than clashes with the olive-green centre; and the tulip tree *Liriodendron tulipifera* 'Aureomarginata', with a butter-yellow edge that fades to lime-green with time, always providing a lovely effect against the deep-green centre. This last is striking both in its individual leaves and as a whole tree. It is unusual to find a *Rhododendron* with variegated leaves, and new cultivars such

When the conifers come into their own

Don't forget winter for foliage colour. This is a time when there is not much colour in the garden, and you can improve the mood with the brighter-hued conifers. The moody blue and serene silver cultivars (such as *Picea pungens* 'Edith' and *Juniperus squamata* 'Blue Star') contrast well with a bit of lively colour from one of their gold relations. Indeed, many of the gold conifers sharpen up their colour in winter, as they dispose of some of their green chlorophyll. They include *Pinus mugo* 'Aurea' and *P. sylvestris* 'Gold Coin'. If you want something gold to intermingle with the prostrate juniper 'Blue Star', try *Abies nordmanniana* 'Golden Spreader', a lovely warm yellow on a frosty day. Don't forget that conifers give off beneficial phytoncides (see pages 172–3), although these chemicals may disperse better on the occasional warmer day in winter.

Silver surfers

Plants with silver foliage can be dramatic in a garden, but you must plan and site them carefully. 'Silver' is a misnomer in some ways, because very few plants have the hue of a knight's breastplate and reflect the light, as true silver does. In reality, such plants tend to fall into grey 'silver' and blue 'silver' foliage types. The former can look dreadfully dreary in midwinter (who needs more grey then?), but the latter, ironically, lift the spirits with their blue sheen. Silver-blue conifers and grasses can be very dramatic, standing resolute against the morning frost.

Where the grey 'silvers' come into their own is on hot, sun-drenched banks. Many Mediterranean plants have grey-silver foliage, so such plants look best in a Mediterranean garden, where their foliage provides a foil to red terracotta or a canopy of bright-pink flowers.

Such images are pleasing to the eye precisely because they mimic the natural landscape. Silver foliage is an adaptation to hot, bright sunlight, a way for plants to protect their vital inner workings by producing pigments or external 'silver' hairs to reflect damaging UV light. Great garden designers recognize that form follows function, in that inspiring designs are intrinsically linked to the ways landscapes and plants actually work, both geologically and ecologically. Essentially, if something functions well, it usually looks right too.

as 'Goldflimmer' and 'Molten Gold' came as a bit of a shock when I first saw them. (My Ph.D involved studying *Rhododendron*, so it is another plant for which I have a soft spot.)

If the variegation is too complex and involves three or more colours, the composition can be confusing. But many gardeners swear by the remarkable *Salix integra* 'Flamingo', its leaves a mix of green, cream and pink – a 'hundreds and thousands' cake-decoration tree if ever there was one.

43 | Let's Be Friends
Talk to your plants

Talking to your plants is good for you and good for them. It is all too easy to forget that plants are living entities. They don't have a brain or central nervous system in the sense in which we understand it, but they are complex living organisms – where different organs within one plant interact effectively, and, indeed, where individual plants communicate with one another and with other organisms. Plants are 'talking' to insects (friends and foes) and their allied micro-organisms all the time. This language is based on chemical signals (very similar to the ways our own cells communicate and organize coordinated responses to a threat or opportunity). In essence, plants have hormones too. Talking to a car when it won't start is just silly; talking to a plant, on the other hand, is perfectly logical.

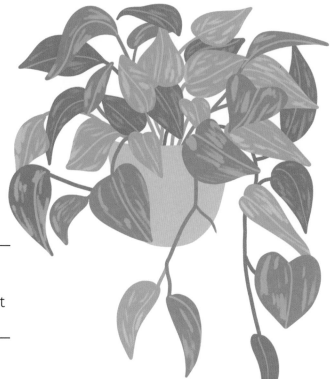

The opportunity to nurture another living being seems important to us

Once we understand that plants are living and want to survive and thrive, our attitudes can change. We are responsible for these living organisms, but that is not as scary as it sounds; the more carefree botanical 'children' need you only to give them a good start in life. Making sure they are planted in soil in a well-lit location and that you supply water for the first few weeks after planting, for example, is all they need – they will do the rest. Those that are more dependent on you (the 'needy' toddlers) – usually those that live in a pot in the living room or bathroom – need more care. You are required to take account of their requirements for light, water and food (fertilizer), and remember to pot them on every so often. If you are talking to your plants, you are probably looking after them really well. You will also be checking that their leaves are deep green and glossy, that no pests (such as scale insects) are annoying them, and that they are not thirsty. You are inadvertently fertilizing them, in that when talking, you are breathing out carbon dioxide – which of course is food for them. You, in turn, are breathing in their chemicals (phytoncides or essential oils) and possibly those beneficial microbiota that help to regulate our physiology (see pages 172–3). So talking really is mutually beneficial.

The opportunity to nurture another living being seems important to us. Feeling needed (even if only by a plant) stimulates positive emotions and perspective, and can be a distraction from woes and worries. Altruistic behaviour is thought to protect against depression and other mental-health problems, although context is important in ensuring a positive response. One thing I have been fascinated by is that in the first week of a new academic year at the university, the sale of houseplants locally increases dramatically as young people, living away from home perhaps for the first time, invest in 'companion' plants. Adding interior decor to a bland university study-bedroom is part of the explanation, I am sure, but perhaps having something to care for provides a degree of security and reassurance too.

44 | **Keep It in the Family**
Learn about the world of phylogeny

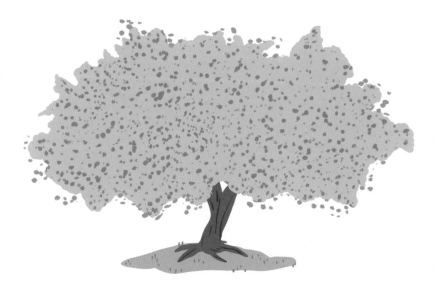

Close inspection of your garden plants will give you clues about where they sit in the bigger 'family tree'

Phylogeny is the evolution of a group of related organisms; their 'family tree'. The phylogeny of plants is fascinating, and understanding it opens up a deeper appreciation of garden plants. This can bring satisfaction and fulfilment, so it is not just the aesthetics of plants that confer positive affect, but also knowledge of them.

What do a buttercup and a delphinium have in common? Not much, you might think. One has plain yellow open, cup-shaped flowers, and creeps around in the lawn. The other has large spires of blue, purple or white flowers, tends to be tall, and is at the mercy of slugs and snails. But the answer is that they are related, botanically speaking; they are both members of the family Ranunculaceae. There are some clues to this. For example, if you look at their leaf patterns, there is some commonality. But most plants are classified taxonomically by flower shape and the number of components within each. Both the wild delphinium and the buttercup tend to have five sepals (green protective coverings for the unfolded flower bud), for example.

Increasingly, genetic profiling is used to identify closely related species. It is more accurate than visual observation, so garden plants are reclassified from time to time. Near cousins become more distant, converting to estranged cousins as it were, and vice versa. We have already seen rosemary being surreptitiously moved from the genus *Rosmarinus* into *Salvia* (see chapter 6).

Close inspection of your garden plants will give you clues about where they sit in the bigger 'family tree'. Some links are obvious. Cherries (*Prunus*) and apples (*Malus*) are both members of the family Rosaceae, for example, and that seems logical when you look at their blossom and the general structure of their fruit, a stone or pip covered with sweet flesh. But the strawberry (*Fragaria × ananassa*) is also in this family, and although its flower conforms to the rules, its seeds (achenes) are on the outside of the fleshy fruit.

Doing this sort of detective work, comparing and contrasting, can be fun. Sometimes the only common feature is the flower shape. Take the Leguminosae (pea family), for example. It comprises tall *Robinia* trees with their rugged, fissured bark; smaller Judas trees (*Cercis*), with smooth bark from which cerise flowers spring directly; thin, wispy brooms (*Cytisus*) bending in the wind; and the toppling flower factories that are sweet peas (*Lathyrus odoratus*). But look closely at their flowers and you will see striking similarities.

Today, we tend to group plants according to aesthetics (colour or size), growing requirements (damp soil, for example) or management criteria (bedding plants being sown and grown together in an annual border). But in traditional botanic gardens the collections were arranged by family, and you can still see some of these plantings in the older botanic gardens.

Health Benefit
Phytoncides (Essential Oils)

Plants produce aromatic compounds known as phytoncides or essential oils that help to protect them from microbial pathogens or herbivorous insects. When we sit quietly in wooded environments, an activity known as 'forest bathing', these chemicals enter our bodies and stimulate certain defence reactions in our physiology, for example activating natural killer cells (lymphocytes) that seek out and deactivate cancer cells.

Forest bathing is a term derived from the Japanese *shinrin-yoku*, 'taking in the forest atmosphere'. It relates to the popular Japanese practice of relaxing, sitting quietly and breathing in the forest air. It was originally thought that the beneficial effects were purely psychological, as people took time to relax and get away from the hurly-burly of life. Only later was a link made between a sense of well-being and some form of biochemical interaction.[18] Researchers started investigating how commonly occurring phytoncides found in the forest – α-pinene and β-pinene, for example – influenced human physiology and the behaviour of cells. It was subsequently found that the enhanced activity of natural 'killer' cells lasted for more than seven days after a forest visit.

This evidence was strengthened by the fact that you don't actually need the trees. In a further experiment, phytoncides were produced in a hotel room by vaporizing oil from the stem of the cypress *Chamaecyparis obtusa* using a humidifier. This corresponded to a significant increase in killer-cell activity, and lower concentrations of the 'fight or flight' hormones (adrenalin and noradrenalin), in those staying overnight.

The phytoncide phenomenon suggests that we are much more closely intertwined with our environment than was previously thought. 'You are what you eat' may be true, but so might 'Your postcode dictates your health', in terms of how the immediate environment determines overall health and well-being. People who live near woodland or other 'wild' areas may have better health prospects because they are more frequently exposed to phytoncides. Add the fact that a number of theories suggest a healthy human microbiome is dependent on regular exposure to the more complex biological communities associated with natural green space, and you see that where we live could have distinct implications for our health. In recent years policymakers have begun to acknowledge this, and they now recognize that there can be significant health inequalities across society, based not simply on income and lifestyle, but also on proximity and access to good-quality and biologically diverse green space.

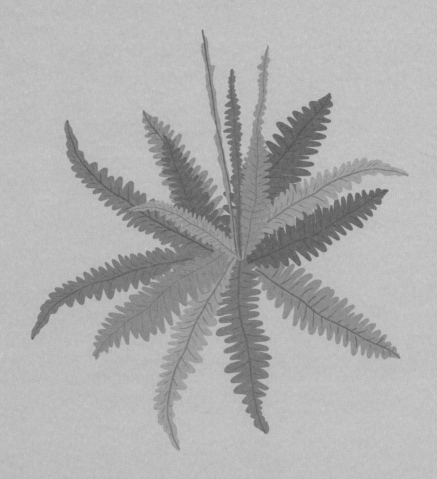

45 | **Eastern Style**
Create a small Japanese garden

Japanese-style gardens are intriguing. As with most things, there is not a simple 'formula' for what constitutes a Japanese garden. Some gardens in Japan are designed to be strolled through, others only to be viewed from a particular vantage point (often a tea house or temple). The latter type are often 'framed' (literally, to represent a picture of the landscape) with bamboo fencing. The minimalist ones, of just a single angular rock and raked gravel, for example, represent a sacred place, and a link to a time when particular rocks in the natural landscape were associated with a divine entity. By contrast, those gardens that contain a greater proportion of plants and water depict the secular world, and deal with more down-to-earth phenomena, such as aesthetics and entertainment. There are commonly occurring themes in both types, however, and many of those induce feelings of calm and order in the viewer.

Many real Japanese gardens borrow scenery from outside the garden itself

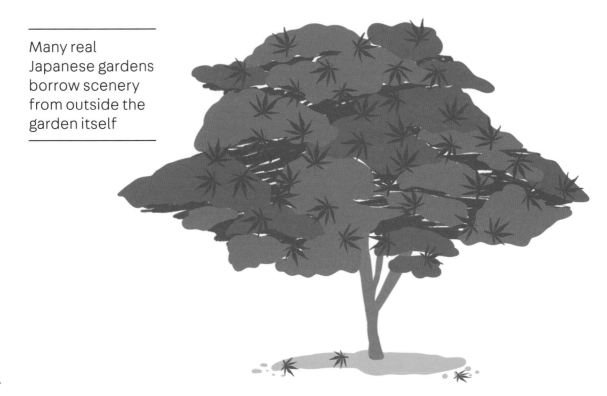

Calming landscapes

Japanese gardens are almost perfect examples of a calm and serene environment. Green spaces in general are seen as calming, and this is no more so than for young people. Even before a baby is born, the environment its mother experiences can have health implications for it. Neighbourhoods with increased tree cover and parkland are linked to increased birthweight. A study carried out on ten-year-olds showed that those living in areas with more greenery had lower (and therefore healthier) blood pressure than those in less green areas, even after accounting for other factors such as temperature, air pollution, noise and urbanization.[19]

Many Japanese gardens symbolize landscapes in miniature (see chapter 46). It may seem paradoxical that these neat and tidy, highly managed garden landscapes are mimicking the wild natural landscapes of Japan (and in some cases China). But such wild landscapes are often idealized; they are the home of spirits, not of untidy humans. A carefully placed rock in a bed of sand or gravel (or perhaps on an island in a more verdant garden) might represent Mount Horai, the mountain home of the immortals. Trees and shrubs will be trimmed to represent different types of forest in scaled-down form. A contorted bonsai might imitate a lonely, wind-blasted pine on the edge of a precipice, while tightly trimmed domed azaleas characterize the bushy canopies of deciduous trees on valley floors. Many real Japanese gardens borrow scenery from outside the garden itself – so if you happen to have a genuine vista of Mount Fuji in the background, so much the better.

Another common feature is to keep aspects of the landscape hidden, allowing them to become apparent only as you move around the garden. This 'hide and reveal' strategy is called *miegakure*. Asymmetry is also important, ensuring that no single feature dominates the scene. A specific feature, such as a rocky 'mountain', should be set off-centre. Using elements in groups of three, but again with irregular sizes and angles, helps to create a natural feel.

Of course, you don't need a degree in Eastern philosophy to create a garden that epitomizes the classical Japanese garden. Take the elements that appeal to you and fashion a tranquil and relaxing space that works for you. You might start with a small pond as a key feature – offset from the middle of your 'picture', of course. On one side plant a Japanese maple (*Acer palmatum*), just to ensure that anyone visiting your garden 'gets' the message. Good forms include 'Beni-maiko', with pink-red foliage unfolding in the spring, and vibrant autumn colour; 'Sango-kaku', with reddish bark for winter interest; and the reliable yet exotic-looking 'Orange Dream'. Slightly more challenging is the full-moon maple (*A. shirasawanum* 'Aureum'). All these will appreciate a spot in partial shade, out of the way of strong wind, and an open, free-draining soil rich in organic matter.

On the other side of the pond, it may be appropriate to situate a moss-covered rock, or perhaps a stone lantern-shaped ornament – in an appropriate Far Eastern vernacular style, of course. If this area is suitably shady, you could encourage the moss on the rock to encroach on to the surrounding ground. You will then end up partaking in the rather unusual activity of weeding grass out of your moss lawn. (Most Western gardeners are animated about removing moss from their grass lawns.) If you fancy the raked-gravel approach, you might use the gravel area to link the pond to a path that runs alongside and behind the pond. Rake the gravel regularly to signify waves lapping against the shore.

In every garden I have owned, I have attempted a few 'cloud formation' trees. This is where you prune a pine or juniper to create balls or clouds of foliage, removing the side shoots and needles completely elsewhere to represent the older trunks, which naturally lose

Forest schools

Forest schools have gained in popularity since the turn of the millennium. They are effectively outdoor classrooms, where children are allowed to learn in natural surroundings. The initiative seems to be particularly beneficial for children who struggle to concentrate in conventional indoor settings. Such woodland settings have, for example, been linked to better management of the symptoms of attention deficit hyperactivity disorder (ADHD), and result in higher academic achievement for such pupils. Even for pupils without special educational needs, green space seems to be beneficial. Improved cognitive development has been noted in children aged seven to ten when exposed to green surroundings, even when factors such as socio-demographics and pollution are taken into account.

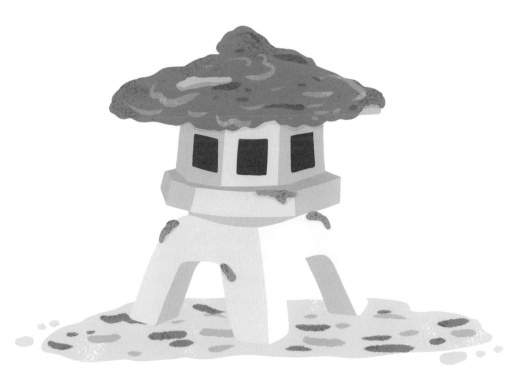

their leaves and branches over time. Good plants to 'play' with
in this way are Scots pine (*Pinus sylvestris*) and Japanese cedar
(*Cryptomeria japonica*). On the subject of 'torturing' plants: regular
trimming of evergreen azaleas (*Rhododendron*) will allow them
to form little baubles of green along a path or interspersed with
carefully placed mountain (rock) outcrops. If you time the pruning
carefully, you may still get a display of flowers in the spring, when
the green bauble turns pink, red or purple, depending on the
cultivar. Trim shoots lightly after flowering, a couple of times if you
can (this will depend on your climate), but avoid trimming after late
summer to ensure that some flower buds form on the new shoots.
Azaleas must have acid soil if they are to grow well, so bear that in
mind when planning.

If space allows, you might include that other horticultural icon of
Japan, the flowering cherry. The one famous for its massed blossom
in Tokyo and elsewhere is *Prunus × yedoensis*, which has flowers that
emerge white (sometimes described as bluish-white), turn pale pink
as they mature and then, just before the petals drop, develop a deep-
rose-pink centre. It eventually forms a spreading, convex-topped

tree. The blossom lasts only two weeks, so this, along with other cherries, represents the fleeting beauty that is revered in Japan. Cherry blossom depicts the concept of *mono no aware* – nothing lasts forever.

The popularity of the cherry in Japan has led to the selection of numerous cultivars over the centuries. The one most commonly found in Western Europe is 'Kanzan', with bronze-green foliage and candy-pink flowers. It is not a bad tree, but its ubiquity has been its downfall to some extent, and it is now dismissed when there are less common cultivars to choose from. My personal favourite is 'Shirotae', with its clusters of polar-white flowers. It is also known as the 'Mount Fuji' cherry, and you can see why, as this lovely tree spreads out into a broad conical shape not unlike the mountain. If you have a serene Japanese pond and want a tree to frame it, this is a great choice, not least because, unlike some other cherries, the leaves remain a fresh green all summer long. 'Tai Haku' ('great white cherry') has similar but larger flowers (hence the 'great'), but it is a much more robust Y-shaped tree and will need space if it is to fulfil its other potential for greatness, as one of the largest cherry trees around. More diminutive and thus better for the small garden is 'Shimidsu Sakura' ('Moon hanging low by a pine tree'), also white-flowered, but with the faintest hint of blue.

The fleeting nature of cherry blossom may give it its cultural symbolism, but it's not ideal in a garden where space is at a premium and where you may want to prolong the period of interest. In that case, *P. sargentii* or *P.* 'Royal Burgundy' are worth considering. Both merit their place on foliage alone; the former turns fiery orange and red in the autumn, while the latter has a deep-purple leaf that turns dark crimson before falling. Both have blush-pink flowers (doubles in 'Royal Burgundy') that provide a super contrast to the dark unfolding foliage in mid-spring.

With the exception of the lotus flower (*Nelumbo nucifera*) – a type of waterlily and a symbol of longevity – the tranquil minimalist philosophy of the traditional Japanese garden is not normally associated with bright summer flowers. However, in a domestic setting I would introduce some 'demure' flowers for no other reason than to maintain seasonal interest. These should resonate with the overall theme, though. One could introduce the elegant shape of Siberian iris (*Iris sibirica*) with its deep-blue flowers at the edge of the pond, or perhaps a bamboo, with its relaxed-looking, hanging foliage (such as *Fargesia murielae* 'Simba'), could be surrounded by a bold drift of Japanese anemones. *Anemone × hybrida* 'Whirlwind', with its double white flowers, is reliable. If you prefer pink, consider *A. hupehensis* var. *japonica* 'Pamina', with double, cup-shaped flowers that appear at the height of summer. Alternatively, *A. rupicola* 'Wild Swan' flowers for longer, if intermittently. Like a wild swan, it is divine, with flowers that are pale grey-blue on the back and pure white on the front.

Where there is a sunny, open spot, the upright stems of herbaceous peonies (*Paeonia*) stand out like ranks of soldiers on parade. Their rigidity is soon challenged, however, as the tight buds morph into magnificent, extravagant floral bowls. *P. officinalis* 'Rubra Plena' is the cottage-garden peony of old, with wine-red blooms. But the herbaceous peony flower also comes as a froth of white (*P. lactiflora* 'Catharina Fontijn'), pink (*P. lactiflora* 'Alertie') and lemon (*P.* 'Bartzella'), or with simpler, single flowers in red (*P.* 'Scarlet Heaven'), white (*P. lactiflora* 'Krinkled White'), pink (*P. lactiflora* 'Nymphe') and lemon (*P. mlokosewitschii*), some with petals set off by a brush of sulphur-coloured stamens.

Finally, don't forget the viewing aspect of your now harmonious landscape. Set up some chairs in the garden to give you a good vantage point, or perhaps design your 'Japanese adventure' so that it can be viewed from a conservatory or living-room window. Either way, make sure you have some tea brewing when friends visit, to complete the experience.

46 | Landscapes in Miniature
Re-create an alpine hillside in a trough

During the COVID-19 pandemic, many people were required to stay at home and could leave their houses only for exercise and to shop for essentials. In an attempt to pass the time and cope with the stress of the situation, they turned to a range of hobbies, including gardening, baking, drawing, painting, learning languages and taking up musical instruments. Many of the activities could be described as 'escapism'. Whether making doll's-house furniture, building model planes (even if the full-sized equivalents were grounded) or creating a rural panorama for an old model train set, many people used their imagination and creativity to switch off and withdraw from the never-ending cycle of negative news.

Common to some of these activities was the idea of seeking sanctuary in a miniature world. This can certainly be done in a gardening context, even in just a few square metres of garden or an old tub or trough. Using appropriate hard materials and plants, you can re-create the Grand Canyon, an alpine mountain range, a dry Arizonan riverbed or a slice of Scottish heather-clad moorland. The knack is to get the plants to look in scale to their surroundings. Grizzled granite boulders can imitate a range of mountain peaks, and sandstone blocks can be used to create a desert cliff face. Gravel or slate chips can mimic montane scree beds, and bits of driftwood play the part of prostrate tree trunks along a dried-out riverbed. Let your imagination run rife – this is your escapist bolthole, after all.

Many plants are naturally dwarf and low-growing because of the harsh environments in which they have evolved. Arctic willow (*Salix arctica*), for example, does not grow more than 30cm (12in) high, even as a 100-year-old 'tree'. To do so would be suicide in the face of

The alpine trough

Many alpine plant specialists use old stoneware troughs or sinks to create their miniature worlds. Such containers are increasingly expensive and hard to come by (never mind the challenges imposed by their weight when moving them). You can, however, make your own rustic trough by covering a much lighter plastic container with hypertufa (a mix of concrete, sand and coir that looks like stone when it hardens). Make sure you insert drainage holes in the bottom of the container, or you may end up with an alpine lake. Fill the trough with gravel, sand or other free-draining aggregates, and place a few rocks to re-create an alpine ridge. Sharply pointed rocks such as granite will give you an arête like the Matterhorn, while more rounded ones (such as sandstone) look like older, weathered mountain ranges such as the Scottish Cairngorms. Align the rocks carefully so that the strata or lines within the rocks line up, as they would in nature. Juxtaposing angles and lines looks distinctly odd; after all, nature has a surprising amount of order in it.

Many people used their imagination and creativity to switch off and withdraw from the never-ending cycle of negative news

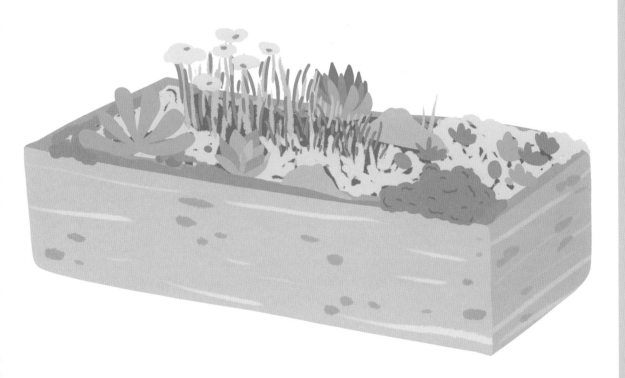

Seeking sanctuary in a miniature
world can certainly be done in
a gardening context

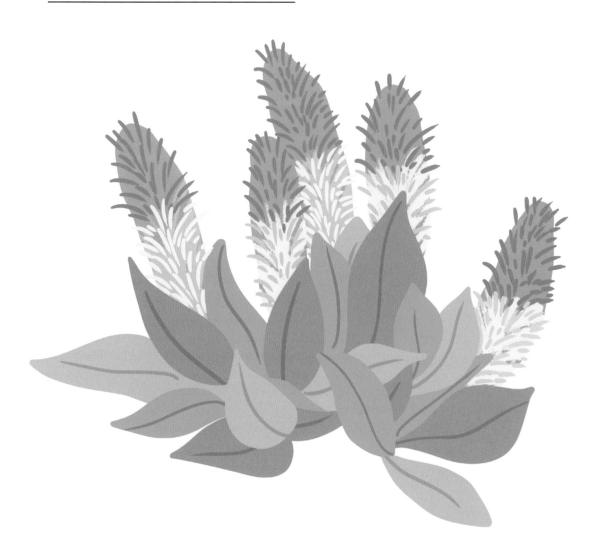

the polar wind. Alpine plants (usually in a dedicated section within garden centres) come with bells, rosettes, panicles or drifts of tiny blooms in yellow, blue, pink or white, but no plant will be more than a few centimetres high and all will be shaped as cushions or mats. Plant these either to re-create an alpine path, or to represent forests in the foothills of your alpine panorama. To my mind the mossy saxifrages, such as *Saxifraga arendsii* 'Scenic Red' and *S. × urbium* (London pride), always look like stands of tropical rainforest seen from a plane. Another saxifrage, the aptly named *S. longifolia* 'Tumbling Waters', looks like a waterfall, with frothy white floral spray tumbling down the 'rockface'.

For the dry riverbed (which could equally represent South Africa or Australia, as well as Arizona), consider growing dwarf grasses among the driftwood. Succulents such as *Delosperma*, *Mesembryanthemum* and the moss roses (*Portulaca*) provide midsummer colour while maintaining the arid theme. The silver-leafed garden *Artemisia* and *Senecio*, such as *A. ludoviciana* 'Silver Queen', can be used to represent the iconic sage brushes of the American Midwest. At the 'drier end' of the river beach you might plunge in some dwarf cacti, such as *Cephalocereus senilis* or *Neocardenasia herzogiana*, to represent their larger Sonoran brethren. Just remember to keep them in their pots, lift them out of the 'riverbed' in autumn and move them indoors for the winter.

Planting for year-round interest

Although a miniature garden is small, it is possible to maintain year-round interest in an alpine trough. A dwarf evergreen conifer or two will be ideal for this. Cultivars of *Pinus mugo* (such as 'Little Delight') tend to be naturally slow-growing and dwarf in habit; other good diminutive types include *Chamaecyparis pisifera* 'White Pygmy', *Picea abies* 'Little Gem', *Pinus heldreichii* 'Smidtii', *Pinus strobus* 'Sea Urchin' and *Abies balsamea* 'Piccolo'. For a blue hue, try *Picea glauca* var. *albertiana* 'Alberta Blue', *Picea pungens* 'Glauca Compacta' or the prostrate *Juniperus squamata* 'Blue Star'. Different forms will suit different situations; *J. communis* 'Miniature' is a good upright form of conifer, whereas *Pinus sylvestris* 'Jeremy' and *Picea sitchensis* 'Papoose' tend to be as wide as they are tall.

For stronger colours in troughs, we are reliant on the dwarf spring bulbs – *Crocus*, *Iris* and miniature species tulips (*Tulipa*) – and on alpine plants themselves. *Aubretia* comes in blues, mauves and occasionally pink, while *Lewisia* ranges across pink, white and apricot. If you have an acid substrate (although please do avoid peat), the gentians (*Gentiana*) can light up the arrangement in a range of light and dark electric-blue flowers.

47 | **Whispering Grasses**
Grow grasses that move with the wind

Before I ever got into gardening, I was always struck by how plants and animals interacted or were affected by the forces of nature. I was fascinated by the way a kestrel could be completely motionless in the sky as it tilted and flexed its muscles against the force of the wind. Trees that grow straight and tall inland would be gnarled and bent when growing by the sea, sculpted by the force of the wind into huddled, hunched, human-like forms about to 'break their backs' in their desperate attempts to avoid the blasts.

Plants and animals are defined by their environment. Plants always seek the light – they are sun junkies – but they also dance to the tune of the wind. Indeed, many plants need wind if they are to be physically strong. Exposure to wind strengthens their cells and promotes secondary thickening, a process that makes the stems more resilient. If you have ever grown a sunflower or other tall

Grasses for relaxation

To experience the relaxing sensation of moving grass, place one or more of the fine-leaved species, such as *Stipa tenuissima* or *Pennisetum setaceum*, in a container or at the edge of a border. Make sure the position is open enough to catch the breeze, and that you can arrange a suitable vantage point – a comfy sofa behind a viewing window will ensure that you drop off to sleep. Where space allows, you could plant a collection of different grasses and rushes. Group them at the edge of a lawn or within a scree bed, or intermingle the grasses with colourful flowering perennials to create a prairie feel.

The different heights, stem strengths and weight of seed heads will allow your grasses to 'express their moods' to the wind in distinctive ways. Species of *Miscanthus* show flexibility while retaining their particular forms, switch grass (*Panicum virgatum*) will sway and twitch with the breeze, and the stiffer, upright stems of bamboo jostle and vibrate against each other as the wind battles to find a passage through. We don't normally think about movement when considering garden plants, but with grasses it is an essential creative component.

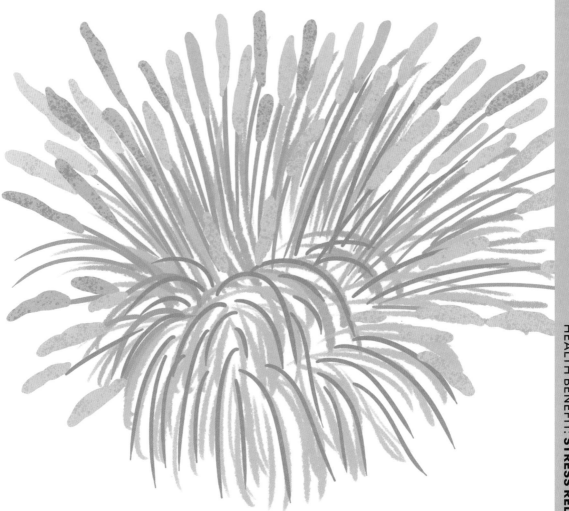

plant in a sheltered greenhouse and then moved it outdoors, you will know what I mean. Within a day or two your lovely straight, proud plant is left battered and broken, while the leftover sunflower seeds you threw on to the vegetable plot have morphed into sturdy, compact and battle-hardened specimens. Plants' interaction with the wind, and the movement and abrasion it causes, is called thigmomorphogenesis (another scientific word that just trips off the tongue).

So plants and the wind have a close interrelationship. Some plants resist the wind: spruces and firs are narrow, columnar trees that let it whistle around them (and the snow slip easily from their sloping branches); and alpine plants hug the ground, forming mats and cushions in the lee of rocks to avoid the full force of the wind. Others

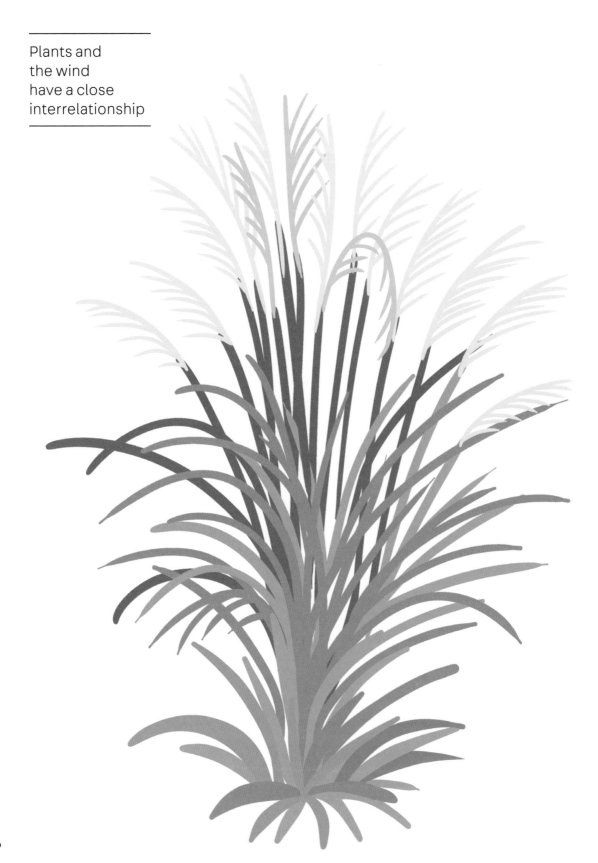

Plants and
the wind
have a close
interrelationship

go with the flow, having flexible stems and leaves. In this second category are the grasses, most of which are open-plain specialists. Depending on their resistance to cold, drought and fire, different grass species constitute different biomes, forming the grasslands of the world: the tundra, steppe, prairie and savannah landscapes. I mention the *inter*relationship between plants and wind because it is a two-way process, since the wind itself is modified by plants. We use plants to provide shelter and create windbreaks, taking advantage of their ability to reduce the force of the wind by absorbing its energy and diffusing its patterns of airflow.

Wind captivates us, as do the other forces of nature: snow, rain and so on. In temperate moods these elements relax us, and we talk about 'gentle breezes', 'soft raindrops', the 'hush of newly fallen snow'. As the energy increases, our emotions move towards exhilaration: 'a blustery, breezy day', 'a wind-blown romance', 'a flurry and blizzard of snow'. At their most extreme, of course, the elements tend to frighten us: 'lashed by the wind', 'caught in a deluge', 'snowed in'. But we are relaxed and exhilarated, too, by the way the wind interacts with plants. Many people love the rustle of leaves, the gentle, rhythmic swaying of branches, the patter of falling seeds, all brought on by temperate air movements. Add energy to the system and we respond in a more excited way: 'trees billowing in a storm' 'leaves cascading across the park in the gale', 'branches clattering against the shutters'.

Ornamental grasses are ideal for reflecting the 'mood' of the wind, and can be used to influence our emotions, too. Soft, fine-leaved grasses swing and sway gently in light breezes. This movement transfixes us and soothes our minds. Every little eddy of the wind is reflected in a gentle twist or upturn of the grass stems or seed heads. I defy you to watch this gentle interplay without unwinding and becoming drowsy. And when the wind drops, the grass relaxes, as though letting out a deep sigh.

48 Spring into Spring
Use early spring flowers

Spring flowers set the new year alight with colour. This is the time when we could all do with a bit of cheer after the long, dark days of winter. The period around 20 January is thought to be the most depressing period of the year for those living in northern latitudes, and the Monday closest to that date is often referred to as 'Blue Monday'. Many of us long for the warmer, brighter days of spring at this time, so the sporadic appearance of flower colour in the landscape shortly after Blue Monday is a genuine boost for morale.

In my garden in East Yorkshire, UK, the pace starts slowly and, as with the increasing daylength, the change is hardly perceptible at first, with the white tips of snowdrops (*Galanthus*) peeking out of the deep-green stems. Similarly, the shy Christmas roses (*Helleborus niger*) hide their beauty, holding their flower heads demurely within last autumn's leaf litter. But with just one brighter day, the unfolding of the petals starts in earnest, almost as if the flower head itself is seeking warmth from the weak winter sunlight. Then the race begins. Before long comes the buzz of the first bee, then the warmer colours of yellow and purple crocuses (*Crocus*), sulphur-yellow aconites (*Eranthis*) and orange, purple and yellow wallflowers (*Erysimum*) all appear in an attempt to flaunt their wares at this unsuspecting insect. As winter begins to wane, we feel genuine warmth in the sunlight again.

An old English adage says that March comes in like a lion (furious) and goes out like a lamb (placid). Whoever said that was obviously talking about the weather, because in the plant world it is precisely the opposite. In early March (or September in temperate parts of the southern hemisphere) we are still in the serene beauty stage, as subtle, pale primroses (*Primula vulgaris*) sprinkle their lovely yellow

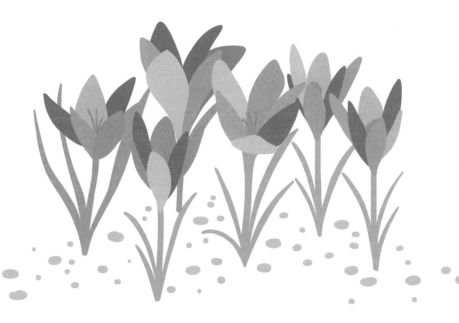

Many of
us long for
the warmer,
brighter
days of
spring

stars among the grass and below trees. A watery-lilac-flowered *Rhododendron* 'Praecox' shelters its blooms from air frosts below the canopy of a spruce tree, and carefully choreographed *Narcissus* 'Ice Follies' flowers uniformly in white and lemon.

Then bang! In my garden by the end of March bright-red, blue, orange, purple, yellow, pink, and pink-and-yellow *Primula* hybrids are escaping and running riot in the borders. The *Narcissus*, too, go crazy, as pinks and vibrant oranges supplant the subtler early hues. Blancmange-pink and ruby-red frilly daisies (*Bellis*) fight it out in the dazzle stakes with purple and orange pansies (*Viola*). Surprisingly – and thankfully – the stronger sunlight seems to let the floral world get away with such effervescent colour. By April, when spring is in full swing, all the plants are throwing caution to the wind. We have the magenta-pinks and blood-scarlets of *Camellia*, and know that the main May battalions of *Rhododendron* and peony (*Paeonia*) are just around the corner.

Whether you appreciate the small, delicate floral harbingers of warmer days, or prefer the tumbling chaos that follows, spring is certainly a time to enjoy. It might arrive tentatively, but before long new life abounds, so take time to notice, and with luck the blues of the dark winter days will be blown away.

49 | Spiritual Rills
Make a short garden rill

By definition, a rill is a small rivulet or brook. In a garden situation it can be straight or naturally meandering, but most are very narrow, as little as 10–15cm (4–6in) wide. The base is impermeable to allow water to flow across the landscape. In more formal rills, the base could be of concrete, stone, coloured tiles or a mosaic of glass beads; essentially any form of lining that is highly ornamental. I remember holidaying in a Portuguese mountain village where the local rivulet was channelled down the high street in a slight depression in the granite cobbles. The rise of the cobbles gave the water a constant rippling effect that caught the light. It was exciting when it rained, because the water rose to about 5–8cm (2–3in) deep, snaking its silvery way downhill and narrowly missing all the front doorsteps.

Rills are used in gardens today to create gentle movement and a relaxing ambience, but the idea of the garden rill goes back a long way. Although they are associated with Islamic gardens, they pre-date the rise of that religion. The earliest were functional, being used in arid landscapes to direct water from a spring to irrigate crops. Water and symmetry were important in early desert gardens, and rills were run at right angles to each other, thus dividing gardens into four equal sections. Designs of this type go back at least to the sixth century BC, with examples associated with the reign of Cyrus the Great in Persia. Early followers of Islam adopted this style and gave it spiritual meaning. Such gardens came to embody the paradise that awaited believers in heaven. The four converging rills represented the four rivers of life, and water in a desert environment was intimately linked with that idea, as the giver and sustainer of life itself. Rills were designed to soothe and to promote spiritual awareness, but they also kept the air cool and discouraged biting insects.

A rill runs through it

A rill can be used to draw attention to a particular feature or act as a link between different parts of a garden. I love the notion of joining a waterspout or downpipe (downspout) from the house to a small garden pond, using a straight rill that runs across the patio. The channel could be sunk below the level of the paving slabs and lined with either attractive tiles (a lovely lapis lazuli hue would be great for that Middle Eastern feel) or deep-green slate sections, fitted over a butyl liner. The joints between the tiles or slates create mesmerizing ruffles and eddies in the flow of water. A pump in the pond recycles water to its source, but additional pipework allows rainwater from the roof to be harvested, keeping the pond topped up naturally. A potted plant or two at either end of the rill will disguise any plastic pipework or visible liner, and deep-blue glazed pots full of azure-flowering *Agapanthus* would be ideal for that purpose.

Rills were designed to soothe and to promote spiritual awareness

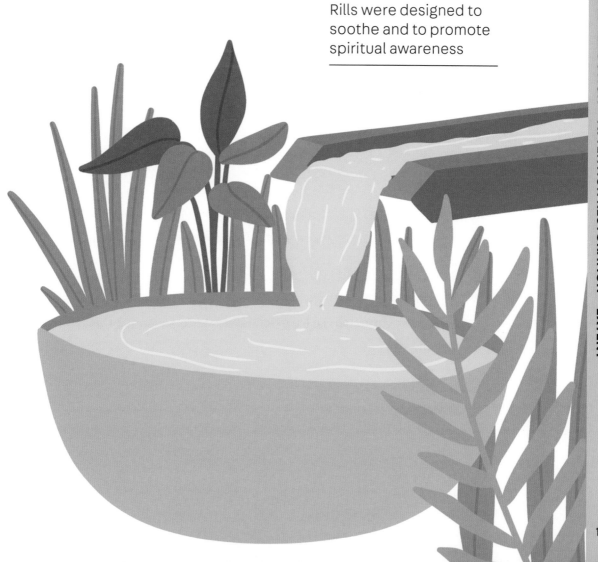

50 | Buzzing Bee Bank
Sow annuals to attract pollinators

Much has been made over recent years of the value of gardens for pollinating insects: bees, butterflies, moths, hoverflies and some beetle species. These insects can be particularly plentiful in traditional meadows, heather moorland, heaths, allotments and around some woodland trees, such as the limes (*Tilia*) and species of willow (*Salix*). They also frequent the flower garden in their search for nectar and pollen. Different insect species have slightly different preferences based on the shape of the flower and the likelihood of getting a reward – nectar – for their visit. There are many perennial flowering plants that support pollinators, but if you don't have a garden, or have only a small plot, consider using annual plants to attract them. Annuals can be grown readily in window boxes, in pots and on balconies.

For bees and other pollinators, we want plants that in the first instance have pollen and nectar. Many ornamental plants have lost these (rather vital) components, or, if they are present, they may be hidden in many folds of petals, and thus not accessible to the insect. For this reason, simple, single annual flowers are usually better than double or multiple-petal forms. A safe bet to provide resources for the bee is to choose plants that have the classic 'cartoon' sun shape – pollen and nectar available in the middle structures, with an array of petals around the edge – as in sunflowers (*Helianthus annuus*), the common marigold (*Calendula officinalis*) and *Cosmos bipinnatus*. Complement these circular flowers with nasturtiums (*Tropaeolum majus*), borage (*Borago officinalis*) and cornflowers (*Centaurea cyanus*). The delicate tracery of baby's breath (*Gypsophila elegans*) adds contrast of form while still providing for the bees.

Bee observant

Take careful notice of your flowers, and you will find that the visiting bees are of more than one species. Most people are familiar with the honeybee and the big bumblebees, but there are other types to look out for. The United Kingdom, for example, supports 127 species, and North America more than 4,000, many of which seem to 'work' for a living. There are mining bees with their furry vertical 'eyebrows'; naturally, they dig holes in the ground. Brown-and-buff-striped plasterer bees are so called because they use a cellophane-like substance to seal their nests. Masonry bees will burrow into any loose joints in a wall, but you could provide them with a bee hotel. In the eastern United States sweat bees don't quite gleam with perspiration, but their metallic thoraxes and abdomens do shine green, blue or black, with greenish-yellow markings. The 'sweat' in their name comes from your hard work, because these species are attracted to salty human sweat. The wool carder bee, meanwhile, will steal the hairs off your plants to line its nest.

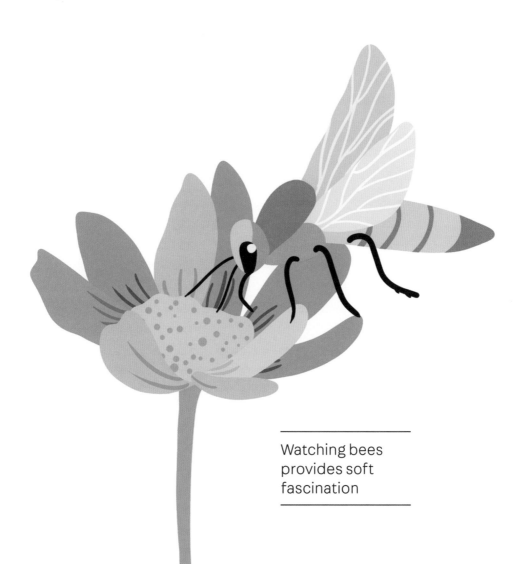

Watching bees provides soft fascination

Add short-lived perennials

If you are gardening in pots and tubs, you can add to the mix of annuals some short-stature, short-lived perennials to boost your 'nectar factory'. Obvious candidates are English lavender (*Lavandula angustifolia*), sages (*Salvia*), speedwells (*Veronica*) and scabious (*Scabiosa* and *Knautia*). You can keep these from one year to the next, but they put so much energy into flowers that they tend not to survive for more than three or four years. Most are readily propagated from divisions (detach some new sideshoots from the base with a bit of root attached) or by taking cuttings.

Watching bees provides soft fascination (see page 123). We become absorbed in their antics as they buzz from flower to flower. The lazy drone of their wings in flight epitomizes the cliché of sunny summer afternoons spent relaxing in the garden. In stark contrast to us, of course, these bees are working hard for a living; no idling on the swing seat with lemonade in hand for them. The honeybee, for example, is an amazingly efficient 'machine' – it can recognize up to 700 different flower aromas, yet to save time it tries to concentrate on one flower type. Because bees must learn how to find the pollen and nectar in each plant species, it makes more sense for an individual to specialize in one flower type that it can 'handle' as quickly as possible. These ladies (workers are female) are doing piecework and must therefore get in and out of each flower as quickly as possible.

In an ideal world, bees would like all flowers to be simple 'sunflower' shapes so that they could be in and out in five seconds. However, it is in the plant's interest for the bee to hang around for longer, because it wants to make sure lots of pollen rubs off on the visitor. Species such as snapdragon (*Antirrhinum majus*) and monkshood (*Aconitum napellus*) have evolved more complex flowers to ensure that the bee stays for longer (up to two minutes in some cases). This seems unfair on the hardworking bee, but there is compensation: these flowers tend to 'reward' the bee with more or richer nectar.

Simple, single annual flowers are usually better for pollinators than double or multiple-petal forms

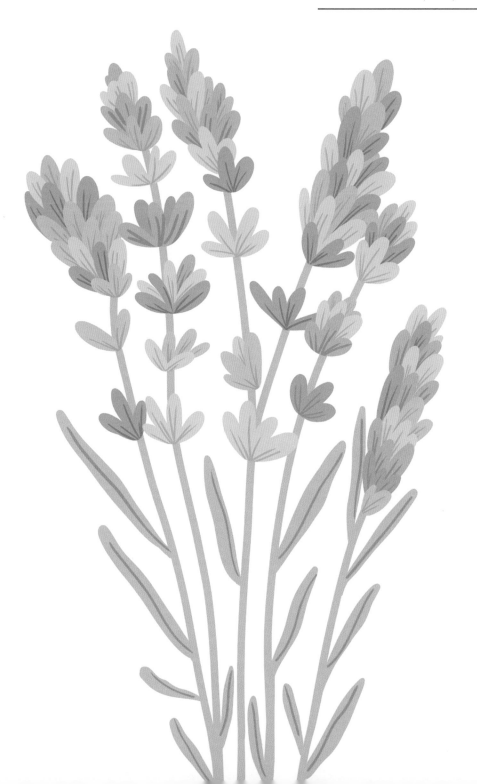

Conclusion

So, can plants save your life? You must make up your own mind. I think they can, although not in the direct, immediate way that a paramedic or surgeon can; plants can certainly prolong life and, perhaps as importantly, improve its quality. For a significant minority they are a key part of life, and make life genuinely worth living.

One of the most compelling theories centres on the idea that for some people, working with and enjoying the presence of plants provide distraction and allow a troubled mind to find a road to recovery. Interventions such as horticultural therapy or green prescribing (outdoor activities including community gardening and the management of wildlife habitat) allow participants to experience non-confrontational environments, find fascination in everyday objects and activities, undertake physical activity (which in itself is a boon for mental health) and acquire a sense of proportion when it comes to the problems with which they are struggling. For some, 'green' activities boost confidence and self-esteem, especially if there is a social element to the activity and constructive feedback, appreciation and friendship are part of the package. In essence, plants (and nature) provide a path to recovery, but perhaps only for some, and it may depend on the sort of mental-health problems or trauma people have actually experienced. The capacity for recovery may also relate to the concept of compatibility, that is to say whether the activity aligns with that individual's values and interests.

This last point may also be the rationale for individuals with an active learning style – those who learn through doing – to gain from these activities, meaning that horticulture is a route into wider educational interests and ultimately better academic achievement. People who find the conventional indoor classroom boring or stressful can excel when their education is centred on a natural environment, as is shown by forest schools, which are particularly valuable in improving the attention span of easily distracted pupils.

Another theory I advocate is that plants and nature provide protection – and this is probably relevant for the majority, not the minority. The more we understand that the human body is essentially a 'city' composed of different organisms and genetic infrastructure, the more the influence of the external environment makes sense. This is where ideas that were until recently considered fanciful are gaining traction. The fact that forest bathing may have some biochemistry to back it up is important. The most obvious example, of course, is what we eat. If we continually throw 'convenient' processed food into our stomachs, rather than foods we evolved with and were 'designed' to eat (berries, fruit, roots and small portions of meat), it is not surprising that we experience health problems. These problems, which relate to unbalanced nutrition, undermine our own gut microbiome, with knock-on effects for inflammatory diseases, immunity and even mental health.

The links between external phytoncides or specific beneficial microbial groups and our health needs further study. There are some compelling concepts, but we need further evidence and to delve into the details of how these compounds or micro-organism groups actually work in terms of promoting health in humans. This is not easy when we consider the large range of microbes that exist, and how they interact with one another and with the wider environment, even before we start to explore how they engage with our own biology and biochemistry. We need a vast amount of information if we are to develop our understanding of the symbiotic relations between humans and micro-organisms. In my world of environmental horticulture, that also means considering the types and quality of green space that people experience, which ones might be particularly beneficial, and why. (This is a current focus of study in my group.)

Despite this requirement for further evidence, there is circumstantial information that supports some of these principles. Not least of these is the fact that, despite our sense of our own sophistication and grandiose ideas about our achievements, culture and 'rightful place' in the universe, we are still a naked ape. What's more, we are one that has been semi-dependent on information technology for as little as 40 years, and on industrial-scale processes for only 300 years. Compare this to 12,000 years of dependence on agriculture and 2.6 million years of hunter-gathering.[20] Although our brains have arguably moved on to suit modern living, our overall physiology is probably still more in tune with hunter-gathering. Thus, logically speaking, it seems strange that we should be so surprised by the benefits of interaction with nature, and our fundamental reliance on it. To me, this is simply common sense.

Plants and gardens have a long history of being therapeutic. Humans in the Paleolithic era would probably have used plants as medicines as well as for food. Although today's pharmaceutical industry has come a long way, it has its roots in herbal medicine and the development of physic gardens in the seventeenth century. There is an irony that the first great industrialists, the Victorians, were also essentially the inventors of the public park, the modern botanic garden and the suburban garden or backyard. They recognized that green space and a love of plants could be a tonic after long hours of toil in the poor working conditions of the 'dark Satanic mills' on which the new wealth depended.

It is also important to remember that gardens are central to many cultural beliefs and religions, being associated with paradise and peace, rest and deeper thought. Many people still feel a spiritual connection to their garden or another green space that they visited and fell in love with. Flowers, of course, are a strong medium for expressing love, gratitude, joy or remembrance.

All in all, then, plants do us good. Indeed, I feel that in this book I have made arguments that plants under certain circumstances can save our lives. This builds on the patently obvious fact that there would not be life as we know it without plants. But we must also recognize plants as ambassadors. The plants you grow in your house or garden are representative of the global biodiversity and integral ecosystems that make life possible in the first place, and we urgently need to value these more and protect them if we ourselves are to survive. By destroying rainforests, damaging ancient woodland, intensifying agriculture, leaving no space for wilderness and inducing climate change, we are 'fraying the wires' of our own life-support system. Plants can save our lives, but let us not squander that opportunity by reducing their chances of survival. Our relationship with plants must work both ways, and be mutual rather than exploitative. So use gardening as a way to explore and appreciate plants and other forms of life in the widest sense. You will be the better for it.

In practical terms this means gardening sustainably, thinking carefully about the resources you might use and where they come from. Do the products you use have a high carbon footprint? If so, think of others and experiment with sustainable alternatives. Go 'green' in terms of energy supply, or go back to manual tools (this is usually better for physical health anyway). The garden should be a place of life, not of chemical extermination. A sterile toilet is one thing, a sterile patio quite another. If you have a pest problem, work to build up natural predators, and avoid pesticides (especially non-selective ones that might damage friend as well as foe).

Remember that the benefits of gardening relate strongly to a certain state of mind, and a mind that aligns with the flows of nature (with some wins and, admittedly, some losses along the way) will be more content. That, ultimately, is the point of gardening: joy and contentment, irrespective of the twists and turns on the journey of plant cultivation.

Text References

All references relate to works listed in the Bibliography.

1. Redondo-Bermúdez et al., 2021.
2. Hirose et al., 2015.
3. Fan et al., 2010.
4. Chalmin-Pui et al., 'Why Garden?'.
5. Cameron et al., 2015.
6. Cameron et al., 2020.
7. Ifeanyi Obeagu, 2018.
8. Chalmin-Pui et al., 'It Made Me Feel Brighter in Myself'.
9. Ulrich, 1984.
10. Cameron and Hitchmough, 2016.
11. Cameron et al., 2014.
12. Cameron et al., 2017.
13. Kaplan, 1995.
14. Robinson et al., 2020.
15. Roslund et al., 2020.
16. Balling and Falk, 1982.
17. Hoehl et al., 2017.
18. Li, 2010.
19. Abbasi et al., 2020.
20. Pretty, 2012.

Bibliography

Behzad Abbasi et al., 'Subjective Proximity to Green Spaces and Blood Pressure in Children and Adolescents: The CASPIAN-V Study', *Journal of Environmental and Public Health* (December 2020)

John D Balling and John H Falk, 'Development of Visual Preference for Natural Environments', *Environment and Behavior*, 14/1 (1982), pp. 5–28

Ross Cameron and James Hitchmough, *Environmental Horticulture: Science and Management of Green Landscapes* (Wallingford, 2016)

Ross Cameron, Jane E Taylor and Martin R Emmett, 'What's "Cool" in the World of Green Façades?', *Building and Environment*, 73 (March 2014), pp. 198–207

Ross Cameron, Jane E Taylor and Martin R Emmett, 'A Hedera Green Façade: Energy Performance and Saving under Different Maritime-Temperate, Winter Weather Conditions', *Building and Environment*, 92 (October 2015), pp. 111–21

Ross Cameron, Jane E Taylor and Emad Salidh, 'To Green or Not to Green! That Is the Question', *Acta Horticulturae*, 1189 (2017), pp. 209–15

Ross Cameron et al., 'Where the Wild Things Are!', *Urban Ecosystems*, 23 (2020), pp. 301–17

Lauriane Chalmin-Pui et al., '"It Made Me Feel Brighter in Myself"', *Landscape and Urban Planning*, 205 (January 2021), p. 103,958

Lauriane Chalmin-Pui et al., 'Why Garden?', *Cities*, 112 (2021), pp. 103–18

Yang Fan et al., 'The Investigation of Noise Attenuation by Plants and the Corresponding Noise-reducing Spectrum', *Journal of Environmental Health*, 72/8 (April 2010), pp. 8–15

Joe Harkness, *Bird Therapy* (London, 2019)

Asuka Hirose et al., 'Tomato Juice Intake Increases Resting Energy Expenditure and Improves Hypertriglyceridemia in Middle-aged Women: An Open-label, Single-arm Study', *Nutrition Journal*, 14/34 (April 2015)

Stefanie Hoehl et al., 'Itsy Bitsy Spider … : Infants React with Increased Arousal to Spiders and Snakes', *Frontiers in Psychology*, 8 (2017), p. 1710

Stephen Kaplan, 'The Restorative Benefits of Nature', *Journal of Environmental Psychology*, 15/3 (September 1995), pp. 169–82

Qing Li, 'Effect of Forest Bathing Trips on Human Immune Function', *Environmental Health and Preventive Medicine*, 15/1 (January 2010), pp. 9–17

Emmanuel Ifeanyi Obeagu, 'A Review on Free Radicals and Antioxidants', *International Journal of Current Research in Medical Sciences*, 4 (February 2018), pp. 123–33

Jules Pretty, *The Earth Only Endures: On Reconnecting with Nature and our Place in It* (Abingdon, 2012)

María del Carmen Redondo-Bermúdez et al., '"Green Barriers" for Air Pollutant Capture', *Environmental Pollution*, 288 (2021), p. 117,809

Jake M Robinson et al., 'Vertical Stratification in Urban Green Space Aerobiomes', *Environmental Health Perspectives*, 128/11 (November 2020), p. 117,008

Marja I Roslund et al., 'Biodiversity Intervention Enhances Immune Regulation and Health-associated Commensal Microbiota among Daycare Children', *Science Advances*, 6/42 (October 2020), eaba2578

R S Ulrich, 'View through a Window May Influence Recovery from Surgery', *Science*, 224/4647 (April 1984), pp. 420–1

Edward O Wilson, *Biophilia* (Cambridge, MA, 1984)

Index

About the Author

The landscape horticulturalist Dr Ross Cameron is research director in the department of Landscape Architecture at the University of Sheffield. Much of his research is into how plants help human society, and he has published over 80 academic papers and contributed to numerous books on landscape plants and urban green spaces. He is co-author of *Environmental Horticulture: Science and Management of Green Landscapes* (2016). As a landscape horticulturalist, he is an advisor to the Agricultural and Horticultural Development Board and the Royal Horticultural Society in the United Kingdom.

Acknowledgements

I am indebted to Romy Palstra for the lovely images that bring this book to life, and to Mark Fletcher, Kevin Hobbs and Kerry Enzor for the original idea and subsequent guidance. Deep thanks are due to those organizations that have provided a forum to discuss the value of plants and gardens and funded research in this area, including the Horticultural Trades Association (Plant for Life), the Royal Horticultural Society, the horticultural therapy group THRIVE, and UK Research and Innovation (Valuing Nature Programme). The book summarizes an amazing amount of hard work, and I would like to thank my fellow researchers, including some whom I have supervised, namely Jo Birch, Tijana Blanusa, Lauriane Chalmin-Pui, Simone Farris, Eun Hye Kim, Veronica Love, Meghann Mears, Madalena Vaz Monteiro, Maria del Carmen Redondo-Bermúdez, Jake Robinson, Emad Salidh, Jane Taylor, Xuezhu Zhai and Liwen Zhang. Lastly, I am grateful to my partner, Gesa, and daughter, Sia, for all those 'spirited discussions' we have about garden management in practice.

First published in Great Britain in 2023 by

Greenfinch
An imprint of Quercus Editions Ltd
Carmelite House
50 Victoria Embankment
London EC4Y 0DZ

An Hachette UK company

A CIP catalogue record for this book is available from
the British Library.

Hardback ISBN 978-1-52942-195-8
Ebook ISBN 978-1-52942-196-5

10 9 8 7 6 5 4 3 2 1

Text by Dr Ross Cameron
Design by John Round Design
Cover and interior artwork by Romy Palstra

Printed and bound in China

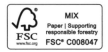

Papers used by Greenfinch are from well-managed forests
and other responsible sources.

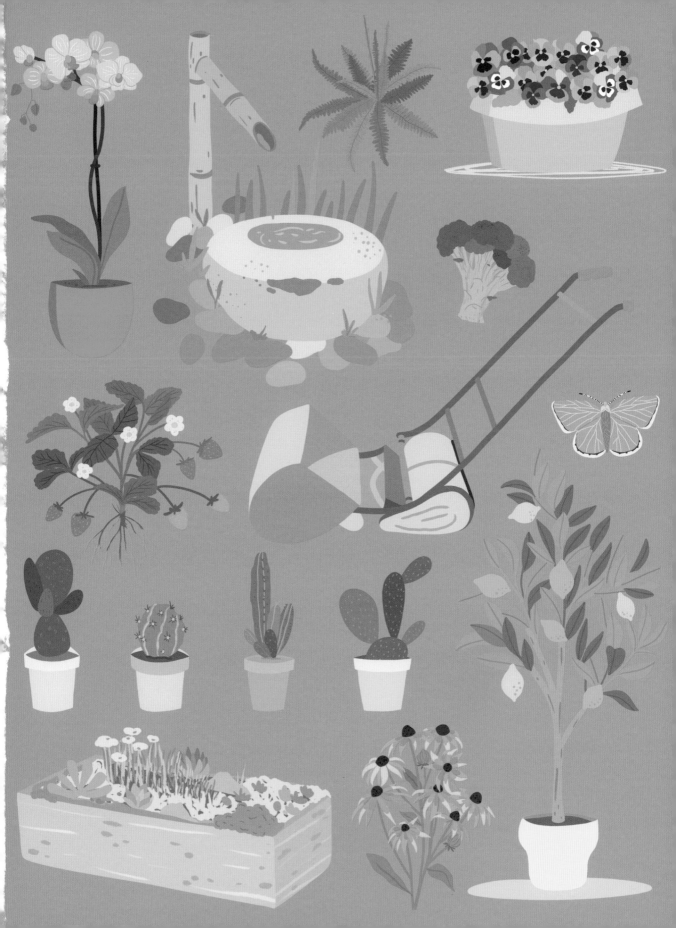

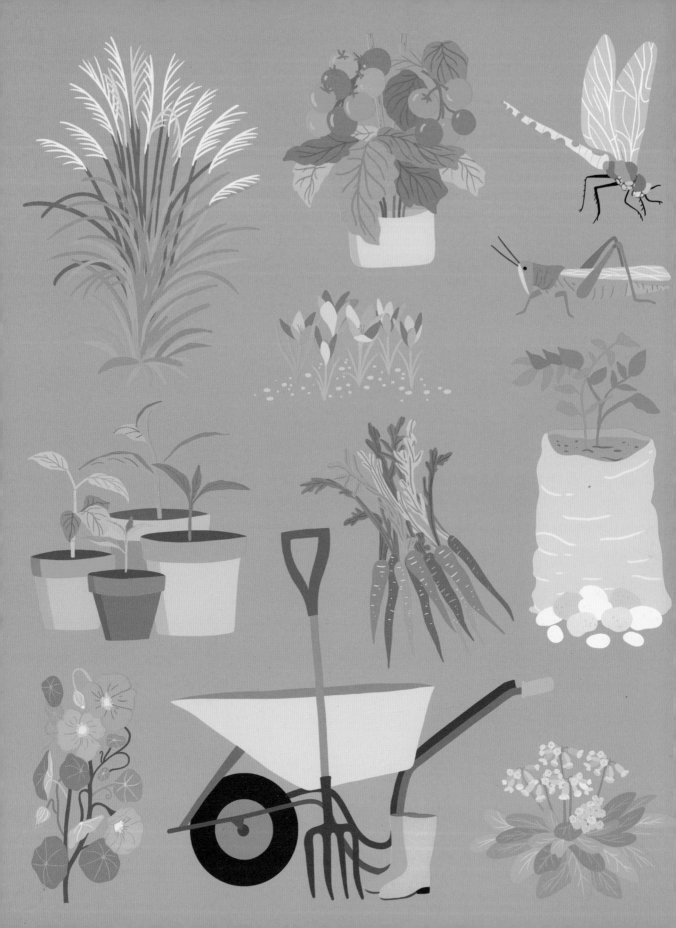